Principal Drugs

An Alphabetical Guide to Modern Therapeutic Agents and Their Use in Some Common Disorders

S. J. Hopkins

Honorary Consultant Pharmacist,

Addenbrooke's Hospital, Cambridge

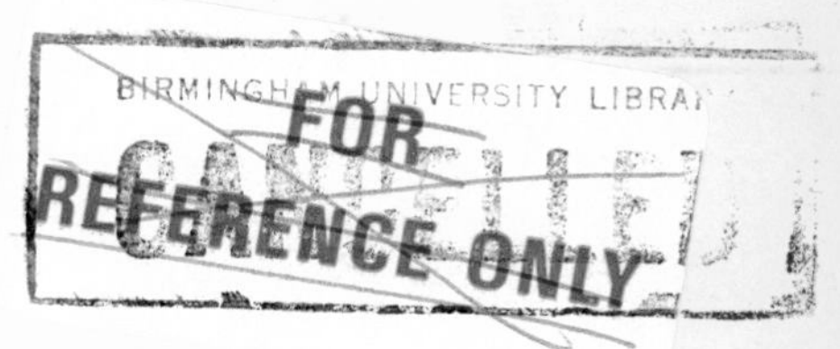

Mosby
Year Book Europe

First published in 1958 by Faber and Faber Limited
3 Queen Square London WC1N 3AU.
Second edition 1964
Third edition 1969
Reprinted 1970
Fourth edition 1973
Reprinted 1975, 1976
Fifth edition 1977
Reprinted 1978
Sixth edition 1980 reprinted 1981
Seventh edition 1983
Eighth edition 1985
Ninth edition 1988
Reprinted 1990

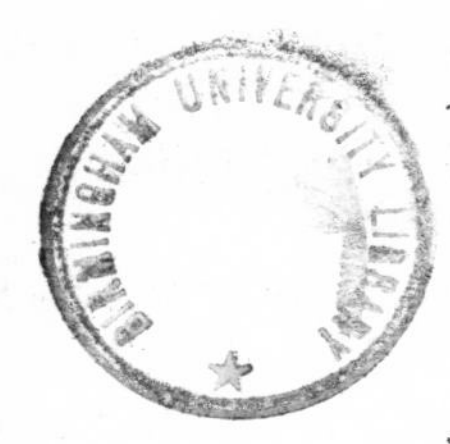

Tenth edition published in 1992 by
Mosby Year Book Europe Limited,
2–16 Torrington Place, London WC1E 7LT.
Photoset by Parker Typesetting Service, Leicester
Printed by Cox & Wyman Ltd., Reading

ISBN 0 7234 1842 X

A CIP catalogue record for this book is available from the British Library.

For a full list of forthcoming titles and details of our surgical, dental and veterinary atlases, please write to
Mosby Year Book Europe Limited, 2–16 Torrington Place, London WC1E 7LT, England.

Contents

Preface

This book, primarily intended for nurses, has now reached its tenth edition, which differs from previous editions in having a new section on the treatment of about 20 common illnesses. In each case, a brief review of the condition is accompanied by an outline of therapy, together with a short list of the main drugs concerned. For further drug information, reference should be made to the Dictionary section of the book. It is hoped that this tenth edition, by giving a concise survey of causes, symptoms and treatment, will clarify the therapeutic pattern and perhaps extend the usefulness of the book to include all those interested in modern drug therapy, whether from the professional or personal point of view.

The Dictionary section follows the pattern of previous editions, but it has been extensively revised, and includes notes on many new drugs, such as alteplase and anistreplase (fibrinolytic agents), imipenem and teicoplanin (antibiotics), enoximone and milrinone (cardiac drugs), ondansetron (a powerful anti-emetic), pravastatin and simvastatin (lipid-lowering agents), vigabatrin (an anticonvulsant), and bone marrow factors, such as erythropoietin and filgrastim. Reference is made to certain groups of drugs, such as diuretics, by tables incorporated in the new text. A few old drugs are included where their continued use warrants their retention. As a rule, no reference is made to mixed products, as these are too numerous, the exceptions being those mixed products recognized by the British National Formulary (BNF), exemplified by co-trimoxazole.

Most drugs are available under a proprietary or brand name as well as under an approved or generic name. The BNF recommends that the latter should be used in prescriptions, and these are therefore used in this book. Extensive lists of both approved and proprietary names are given on pages 221–266. As those lists refer to some drugs not included in the text, an indication is given of the nature of the drug or its action, so that reference back to similar drugs described in the Dictionary section may be possible.

The doses given in this book are for guidance only. For confirmation before using a drug, and for further information, reference should be made to official publications, such as the *British National Formulary* and *Martindale's Extra*

Pharmacopoeia, or to the literature issued by the manufacturer of the product concerned.

The publisher, in this edition, has used the international standard in abbreviating micrograms to μg. Readers should be aware that it is recommended that micrograms should be written out in full in all prescriptions.

Thanks are due to those readers who have commented on the book or suggested alterations, and a note of any errors or omissions will be appreciated.

S.J.H. 1992

Notes on dosage

In this dictionary of drugs the doses, unless otherwise stated, are average daily doses for adults, and are normally given as divided doses at suitable intervals. An indication is given of those few drugs that are taken as a single daily dose, or where the dose is based on the surface area of the body expressed as square metres (m^2). When a dose range is indicated, a small initial dose is often followed by gradually increasing doses according to need and response, but with long-acting drugs, care must be taken to avoid excessive dosage, as such drugs may then accumulate in the body and have toxic side-effects. It should be noted that the side-effects of a drug may prevent the administration of an optimum therapeutic dose, and a recommended dose is often a compromise between activity and toxicity.

Dosage is also influenced by the route of administration, as oral doses are normally larger than those given by intramuscular injection, and the latter are in turn larger than those given intravenously. The weight, age and sex of a patient may also have to be taken into account when assessing dosage. Renal and hepatic impairment may require an adjustment of dose, whereas if tolerance to a drug develops, a larger dose may be required to evoke an adequate response. Dosage also requires particular care during pregnancy if toxic effects on the fetus are to be avoided and, ideally, no drug should be given in pregnancy unless the need outweighs the risks.

Doses for infants also present problems. Their drug-detoxifying enzyme systems and renal excretory capabilities are not fully developed although, paradoxically, they have higher metabolic rates than adults, and so may sometimes require an apparently relatively high dose of a drug. Many schemes for basing children's doses on body-weight, or body-weight plus age, have been described, but doses based on surface area of the body are now considered more reliable. Taking the body-surface of an average adult to be 1.8m^2, the approximate dose of a drug for a child can be expressed as a percentage of the adult dose:

$$\frac{\text{surface area of patient as } m^2}{1.8} \times 100 = \text{per cent of adult dose}$$

(See **Table 1**)

Doses for the elderly also frequently require modification, as their reduced renal efficiency may cause accumulation of the drug and increase susceptibility to toxic effects, unless reduced doses are given. Elderly patients are, in any case, more susceptible to nephrotoxic drugs generally. Hepatic disease may also increase drug toxicity as liver enzymes play a major part in drug metabolism and severe liver disease may give rise to a drug toxicity that might not otherwise occur. Hyperlipidaemic drugs, fusidic acid and some penicillin esters of the talampicillin type are examples of drugs best avoided in hepatic disease. Multiple therapy may also lead to an increased and not always appreciated incidence of drug toxicity. For further information on these important aspects of drug dosage, a book for nurses on drugs and pharmacology should be consulted.

Table 1. Estimating children's doses (*expressed as a percentage of the adult dose*)

Age	Body surface (m^2)	% of adult dose
2 months	0.28	15
4 months	0.36	20
6 months	0.4	22
12 months	0.49	25
3 years	0.65	33
7 years	0.88	50
12 years	1.25	75

Drug administration and responsibility

Nurses should remember that the responsibility for drug administration is delegated to them by doctors, and that they act under medical direction. There is a trend to extend nurses' responsibilities to certain aspects of drug administration that are normally dealt with by medical staff, and nurses should be clearly aware for what they are accountable, and where their responsibility ends.

Before any drug is administered, the name of the drug and the dose should be checked with the prescription and the product. The golden rule is READ THE LABEL. If there is any doubt whatsoever, confirmation with a senior officer should be sought. **Belief** that the correct drug in the correct dose has been given is no substitute for certainty. Nurses are responsible for any errors that they may make, and must be prepared to accept the full consequences.

Controlled drugs

Drugs likely to cause dependence and misuse are referred to as 'controlled drugs', as they are subject to the strict prescription requirements of the Misuse of Drugs Act, 1971, and are distinguished in this book by a dagger †. They include opium, morphine, heroin (diamorphine), pethidine and other synthetic, potent analgesics/narcotics, dihydrocodeine injection, barbiturates (except intravenous anaesthetics) and amphetamines. Controlled drugs can be supplied only on receipt of a hand-written prescription from the prescriber, giving full details of the patient, the drug, the form and strength of the prescription to be dispensed, and the total amount to be supplied expressed in both words and figures. Certain weak preparations of some controlled drugs, such as Chalk and Opium Mixture for diarrhoea, with which misuse is unlikely, are exempt from control, and can be obtained without prescription.

Drug compliance

An increasing problem of current therapy is patient compliance with prescribed treatment. It is easy for a doctor to prescribe, but to ensure that the patient takes the prescribed drugs in the right dose is a very different matter. The magnitude of the problem has increased with the rise in multiple therapy, and the reluctance on the part of some doctors to prescribe mixed products so that the number of different tablets or capsules to be taken daily can be reduced. It must be admitted that relatively few patients leave the consulting room with a clear idea of the nature and dose of the prescribed medication, partly as a result of fear of the doctor, and partly because of the difficulties of understanding complex therapy.

Here, nurses can play a valuable part in reducing difficulties and misunderstandings, particularly when dealing with the elderly and/or confused patient, and it is often helpful to ask a patient to repeat the directions that they believe they have been given. Misunderstandings and errors can then be cleared up at an early stage. The containers of the dispensed medicines should not only bear the name of the drug, but also useful additional information such as 'The Heart Tablets' or 'The Water Tablets'. Vague directions should be avoided: whenever possible definite times for administration of drugs should be arranged. Such timing can be linked with some regular activity, such as a meal time, or a favourite TV programme may be used as a memory aid for regular dosing. With multiple therapy, patients should be encouraged to set each day's dose aside, so that a double dose of a drug will not be taken by forgetfulness. Patients should be advised that the occasional missed dose is not always important, and a missed dose should *not* be made up by taking a double dose later on.

Although regular dosing is important in securing patient compliance, many modern drugs have relatively long half-lives so the regular administration of full doses for long periods may lead to overdose. The ideal dose depends on many factors, including absorption, metabolism, transport and excretion, but in many cases the margin of safety is fairly wide. In the elderly, however, reduced renal efficiency may lead to the gradual accumulation of a drug with insidious toxic effects. Many elderly patients, for example, on digoxin, may become over-digitalized because of poor metabolism and excretion of the drug. It is by no means unknown for elderly and confused patients, once admitted to hospital for observation, to make an apparently surprising recovery from an illness that was basically due to over-medication, often as a result of following blindly a misunderstood drug regimen. It is here that the community nurse has an exceptionally valuable part to play in ensuring regular and accurate medication, and reporting any incipient signs of overdose or side-effects.

The Committee on Safety of Medicines has a 'yellow card' system for physicians to report on reactions that may occur with recently introduced drugs.

Dictionary of drugs

A

ACE inhibitors *See* angiotensin-converting enzyme inhibitors.

acebutolol A beta-adrenergic blocking agent with the actions, uses and side-effects of propranolol, but with a more cardio-selective effect and less likely to cause bronchospasm. *Dose:* in hypertension, 400–800mg daily; in angina, up to 1.2g daily. In severe arrhythmias, acebutolol may be given by slow intravenous injection in doses of 25mg. It is contra-indicated in cardiogenic shock, atrioventricular-block and heart failure. Care is necessary in obstructive airway disease and renal failure.

acetazolamide An inhibitor of the enzyme carbonic anhydrase that has been given as a mild diuretic, as it increases the excretion of bicarbonate. It is now used mainly in mild glaucoma, as it decreases intra-ocular pressure by reducing the formation of the aqueous humour. It has also been used for *petit mal. Dose:* 250mg–lg daily. In severe conditions it may be given in similar doses by intravenous injection. Side-effects are drowsiness, gastrointestinal disturbances and paraesthesia.

acetic acid The weak acid present in vinegar. Acetic acid, well diluted, has been used as a cooling lotion, and a 0.25% solution has been used for bladder irrigation.

acemetacin A derivative of indomethacin with similar actions and uses, but said to be better tolerated. *Dose:* 120–180mg daily.

acetomenaphthone A synthetic vitamin K, formerly used in prothrombin deficiency. Menadiol and phytomenadione are now preferred. Acetomenaphthone is present in some chilblain preparations.

acetylcholine The neurotransmitter of the parasympathetic nervous system. A 1% solution is sometimes used as a miotic to obtain rapid contraction of the pupil after cataract surgery.

acetylcysteine A mucolytic agent used to reduce the viscosity of pulmonary secretions in respiratory disorders and cystic fibrosis. *Dose:* direct instillation of a 20% solution of 1–2ml every 1–4 hrs; by nebulization, 2–5ml three or four times a day; orally, 600mg daily in acute and chronic bronchitis. It is also of value in the *early* treatment (10–15 hours) of paracetamol poisoning with an initial dose of 150mg/kg by slow intravenous injection, followed by smaller doses up to a total dose of 300mg/kg over 20 hours. It is ineffective, and possibly harmful if given at a later stage.

acetylsalicylic acid Aspirin, *q.v.*

acipimox A derivative of nicotinic acid used in hypercholesterolaemia. *Dose:* 500–750mg daily. Side-effects are flushing, erythema, nausea and malaise.

aclarubicin An anthracycline cytotoxic agent used in resistant acute non-lymphatic leukaemia. It is given by intravenous infusion in doses based on skin area and the patient's condition, with monitoring of cardiac function. The side-effects are those of related drugs. *See* doxorubicin.

acriflavine An orange-red dye with antiseptic properties. It was once used extensively as a lotion (1:1000).

acrivastine One of the newer antihistamines. It is less likely to cause drowsiness, as it does not cross the blood-brain barrier to any great extent, but is correspondingly less effective in non-allergic pruritus. *Dose:* 24mg daily.

acrosoxacin A synthetic antibacterial agent of the ciprofloxacin group, with similar side-effects. It is used in penicillin-resistant gonorrhoea as a single dose of 300mg.

ACTH *See* corticotrophin.

actinomycin D A cytotoxic antibiotic, also known as dactinomycin, that inhibits cell division by forming a stable complex with DNA. It is used mainly in Wilm's tumour, and tumours of the uterus and testes. *Dose:* 500μg daily for 5 days by intravenous infusion; but other dosage schemes are in use. It is highly irritant to soft tissues, and great care must be taken to avoid extravasation. Close haematological control is necessary. Skin eruptions, alopecia and gastrointestinal disturbances are frequent side-effects.

acyclovir An antiviral agent highly active against herpes simplex and zoster viruses. It acts indirectly by inhibiting the DNA polymerase essential for viral replication. *Dose*: 200mg five times a day for 5 days in herpes simplex infections of the skin and mucous membranes, and in genital herpes: in shingles (herpes zoster), 800mg orally five times a day for 7 days is given, but treatment should be started as soon as possible to obtain the maximum relief of pain. A 5% cream is used for superficial infections, and for herpes simplex keratitis a 3% ophthalmic ointment is available. Acyclovir is also of great value in herpes simplex infections in immunocompromised patients. *Dose:* 200mg four times a day; 800mg five times a day in zoster infections. In severe conditions, 5mg/kg, or more, 8-hrly by intravenous infusion. It is also given orally for long-term prophylaxis in such patients. Reduced doses are necessary in renal impairment and in the elderly. Side-effects include gastro-intestinal disturbances, rash and neurological reactions.

adenosine A cardiac drug that slows conduction through the AV node. It is used to restore normal sinus rhythm in paroxysmal tachycardia, given by rapid intravenous injection as an initial dose of 3mg. A second dose of 6mg may be necessary after 1–2 minutes, and a third dose of 12mg if the tachycardia remains uncontrolled. For use only with close cardiac monitoring. (*Note:* adenosine phosphates play an important part in cell energy exchange).

adrenaline Known in the US as epinephrine, adrenaline is one of the principal hormones of the medulla of the adrenal gland, but is now made synthetically. It acts on both the alpha and beta receptors of the sympathetic nervous system. The effects on the alpha receptors result in vasoconstriction with a rise in blood pressure; stimulation of the beta receptors increases cardiac rate and output, and relaxes bronchial muscles. *Dose:* in acute bronchospasm, 0.2–0.5ml of 1–1000 solution by subcutaneous or intramuscular injection. In anaphylactic shock and allergic emergencies, 0.5–1mg (0.5–1ml of 1 : 1000 solution) is given by intramuscular injection and repeated every 15 minutes as required. An intravenous injection of an antihistamine is sometimes given as supportive therapy. Doses of 100–200μg (1–2 ml of 1 : 10 000 solution) have been given by intracardiac injection in cardiac arrest and syncope. In hypotensive crises, noradrenaline or metaraminol, are preferred. It is added to local anaesthetic solutions (1 : 50 000–1 : 200 000) to prolong the anaesthetic effect by reducing diffusion of the anaesthetic solution. Occasionally the solution is applied locally to stop capillary bleeding and epistaxis. It is also used as eye-drops (1%) in glaucoma. Solutions of adrenaline may darken on storage and lose activity.

albumin (human) Human albumin, obtained from pooled human plasma, is given by intravenous infusion as a 5–20% solution in the treatment of shock and other conditions where restoration of blood volume is urgent; in severe burns to prevent haemoconcentration, and in some conditions of hypoalbuminaemia, and in acute oedema.

alclometasone. A highly potent topical corticosteroid. It is used as a 0.05% cream or ointment in inflammatory and pruritic dermatoses likely to respond to such therapy. Contra-indicated in infected skin lesions, and prolonged therapy should be avoided.

alcohol (ethanol) Used occasionally by injection to destroy nerve tissue in the treatment of intractable trigeminal neuralgia. Industrial alcohol or methylated spirit contains 5% of wood naphtha; surgical spirit is industrial spirit with the addition of methyl salicylate and other substances and is used for skin preparation and the prevention of pressure sores. Ordinary, coloured, methylated spirit contains pyridine, and is not suitable for medical purposes.

alcuronium A muscle relaxant similar to tubocurarine, but more powerful. It causes less histamine release but some transient fall in blood pressure may occur. *Dose:* 10–15mg intravenously, and subsequently 3–5mg as required. Sensitivity to alcuronium is increased by inhalation anaesthetics, beta-blocking agents and aminoglycoside antibiotics. The action can be terminated by the intravenous injection of neostigmine.

aldosterone The main mineralocorticoid hormone of the adrenal cortex. An excessive secretion of aldosterone may occur in some oedematous states and reduce the action of thiazide diuretics. See spironolactone and canrenoate.

alfacalcidol A derivative of calciferol, with a more powerful and rapid action. It is used to treat hypocalcaemia in hypoparathyroidism, neonatal hypocalcaemia and other hypocalcaemic states, and in vitamin D-resistant conditions. Regular blood calcium determinations are essential as a drug-induced hypercalcaemia may take weeks to subside after withdrawal. *Dose:* 1μg daily, initially, according to response.

alfentanil A potent, rapidly acting narcotic analgesic, useful in short surgical procedures, or for longer operations in ventilated patients. The peak effect occurs about 90 seconds after intravenous injection, with recovery after 5–10 minutes. *Dose:* 500μg i.v., initially, followed by 250μg as required.

alkylating agents Cytotoxic drugs which act by damaging DNA, and so interfere with cell replication. Chlorambucil, and cyclophosphamide are examples.

allergen vaccines Weak allergen vaccines prepared from allergens such as grass pollens, house dust mites and bee stings are used to desensitize hypersensitive individuals, but the results are not always satisfactory. Such treatment carries the risk of severe anaphylactic reactions, which may prove fatal in asthmatics, and it is now recommended that desensitization therapy should be carried out only when full cardiorespiratory resuscitation measures are immediately available.

allopurinol An enzyme inhibitor that blocks the formation of uric acid, and so is useful in the treatment of chronic gout. It also reduces the risk of uric acid calculi. It is useful in the hyperuricaemia of leukaemia but it should be given before cytotoxic therapy is commenced. *Dose:* 100mg daily as a single dose with food, slowly increased to 300mg daily or more as required, reduced in cases of renal impairment. It may cause gouty arthritis initially, requiring colchicine or NSAID treatment for at least one month. Side-effects include nausea, headache and gastro-intestinal disturbances, but skin reactions indicate withdrawal of the drug.

allyloestrenol An orally active progestogen with few side-effects. *Dose:* in threatened abortion 15mg daily; in habitual abortion 5–10mg daily as soon as pregnancy is diagnosed, and continued as necessary.

almasilate Aluminium magnesium silicate. An antacid with the actions, uses and doses of hydrocalcite.

aloxiprin Aspirin in combination with aluminium oxide. It has the actions and uses of aspirin, but causes less gastric irritation. *Dose:* up to 4.8g daily.

alprazolam A benzodiazepine used in the short-term treatment of anxiety and anxiety with depression. *Dose:* 0.75–3mg daily. Side-effects include dizziness and ataxia. Care is necessary in pulmonary insufficiency.

alprostadil A preparation of prostaglandin E_1 for intravenous use in maintaining the patency of the ductus arteriosus in neonates with congenital heart lesions requiring surgical correction. The improvement in circulation so obtained permits diagnosis while surgery is being considered. *Dose:* 0.1μg/kg per minute under strict control. Apnoea may occur, usually within an hour of the injection, requiring immediate ventilatory assistance. Bradycardia and hypotension may also occur.

alteplase A form of human plasminogen activator with a selective fibrinolytic action on blood-clot-bound plasminogen. It is of value in the *early* treatment (6 hours) of acute thrombosis and myocardial infarction. *Dose:* 10mg initially by slow intravenous injection; then 90mg over 3 hrs by intravenous infusion. Side-effects are nausea, vomiting and local bleeding. See streptokinase.

alum Used for its astringent properties as a mouthwash and as a lotion, 1–2%. Weak solutions have been used for bladder irrigation.

aluminium The powdered metal is used as a skin protective in ileostomy, as Baltimore paste, also known as Compound Aluminium Paste.

aluminium acetate An astringent used as an 8% solution for ear-drops in otitis externa. A weak solution (0.65%) is used as a lotion in exudative eczematous states and in suppurative conditions.

aluminium chloride An antiperspirant used in the treatment of axillary hyperhydrosis by the local application of a 20% alcoholic solution. Overuse may cause skin irritation.

aluminium hydroxide An antacid with a prolonged action. Unlike the carbonates, it does not liberate carbon dioxide, is not absorbed and so does not cause alkalosis. *Dose:* Given in suspension as a gel, 7.5–15ml, or as 500mg tablets, to be chewed or crushed before swallowing.

alverine An antispasmodic with a local action on intestinal smooth muscle. Used in irritable bowel syndrome in doses of 60–360mg daily.

amantadine An antiviral drug thought to act by inhibiting the penetration of the virus into the host cell, and used for the prophylaxis and treatment of influenza. It is also used with levodopa in the treatment of parkinsonism, but it may relieve the rigidity more than the tremor. *Dose:* 200mg daily. Many side-effects are dose-related.

amethocaine hydrochloride Powerful local anaesthetic, used for anaesthesia of mucous membranes 1–2% solution, eye-drops 0.25–1%. As spray for throat before endoscopy, etc., 0.5% solution may be used. Hypersensitivity and allergic reactions may occur as with other local anaesthetics.

amikacin A semi-synthetic antibiotic similar in actions and uses to kanamycin, *q.v.* Mainly used in the short-term treatment of serious infections due to Gram-negative, gentamicin-resistant organisms. *Dose:* 15mg/kg daily by i.m. injection or intravenous infusion, up to a total treatment dose of 15g. Side-effects include ototoxicity, drug fever, rash and nausea. Dose should be reduced in renal impairment.

amiloride A potassium-conserving diuretic with an action on the distal tubule similar to that of spironolactone, although it is not an inhibitor of aldosterone. It is used in hypertension and heart failure, often with a thiazide diuretic to obtain a more balanced response. *Dose:* 5–20 mg daily. Rash is an occasional side-effect.

amino acids Certain amino acids are essential for the formation of protein. When oral nutrition is not possible, amino acid preparations may be given by intravenous infusion, and such therapy can be extended if necessary to provide total parenteral nutrition by the addition of glucose, electrolytes, fats and vitamins as specially prepared solutions. For long-term therapy in hospitals, a 24-hour supply for total parenteral nutrition can be provided in a single large container. Patients may be taught to administer total parenteral nutrition at home. Representative amino-acid products for intravenous infusion are Aminoplex, Perfusin, Synthamin and Vamin.

aminobenzoic acid An absorbent of some of the erythema-producing ultra-violet light waves of sunlight. It is used as a 5% solution as a sunscreen, but the action is brief, and frequent application of the solution to the skin is necessary in extended exposure to sunlight.

aminoglutethamide An inhibitor of adrenal steroid and oestrogen biosynthesis. It is used in the control of post-menopausal oestrogen-dependent mammary carcinoma and in the treatment of advanced prostatic carcinoma. *Dose:* 500mg daily, increased, if necessary, to 1g daily. Supplementary corticosteroid therapy is essential. Side-effects include drowsiness, rash and drug-fever.

aminoglycosides A group of antibiotics that includes amikacin, gentamicin, netilmicin, tobramycin, kanamycin, streptomycin, neomycin and framycetin. They act mainly against Gram-negative bacilli, although they are also active against some Gram-positive organisms. Kanamycin and streptomycin are also active against *Mycobacterium tuberculosis*. The aminoglycosides are not absorbed orally and in systemic infections they must be given by injection. They are more toxic than most other antibiotics, and in renal impairment care is necessary, as the plasma concentration of the antibiotic may rise to an ototoxic or nephrotoxic level. The toxicity may also be increased by diuretics of the frusemide type. Measurement of plasma levels is essential in high dosage or continued therapy. Gentamicin is the most widely used aminoglycoside for systemic infections, and neomycin and framycetin, being too toxic for systemic use, are of value in skin infections.

aminophylline A derivative of theophylline with a similar bronchodilator action. It is used chiefly in asthma, cardiac oedema and congestive heart failure. *Dose:* 300mg–1.2g orally daily; 5mg/kg may be given by *slow* intravenous injection. It is not suitable for intramuscular administration. A sustained-release oral product is available that causes less gastric disturbance.

amiodarone An iodine-containing anti-arrhythmic agent of value in all types of paroxysmal tachycardia, especially when the condition is resistant to other drugs. *Dose:* 600mg daily for one week; maintenance, 200mg or less daily. When a rapid response is required, 5mg/kg may be given by intravenous injection under cardiac monitoring. It is contra-indicated in bradycardia, pregnancy and thyroid disorders, and care is necessary in hepatic impairment. Pulmonary alveolitis, corneal microdeposits and photosensitivity have been reported as side-effects.

amitriptyline A tricyclic antidepressant similar in action to imipramine, but it also has anxiolytic and sedative properties. *Dose:* in depression complicated by anxiety, 30–150mg daily initially; maintenance, 20–100mg daily; sometimes as a single nightly dose to reduce daytime sedation. Lower doses are often adequate in elderly patients. By injection, 40–80mg daily. Full benefit may not be achieved for some weeks and prolonged therapy may be necessary to avoid relapse. Withdrawal of the drug should be gradual. Amitriptyline is also used in nocturnal enuresis in children. *Dose:* 25–50mg daily. Side-effects include dryness of the mouth, sedation and cardiac arrhythmias. It is contra-indicated in glaucoma, prostatic hypertrophy and after recent myocardial infarction.

amlodipine A calcium channel blocking agent used in hypertension and myocardial ischaemia associated with angina. *Dose:* 5–10mg daily. Side-effects are headache, dizziness, flushing and oedema. Care is necessary in renal impairment.

ammonium chloride A mild expectorant and diuretic; has been given in association with mandelic acid in urinary infections. *Dose:* 300mg–2g daily.

amorolfine An antimycotic used in the treatment of fungal infections of the nails. It is applied to the nails as a lacquer (5%), but prolonged treatment at weekly or twice weekly intervals for some months is required until the nails are regenerated.

amoxapine A tricyclic antidepressant with the actions, uses and side-effects of imipramine, but giving a more rapid initial response. *Dose:* 100–250mg daily, with half-dose for elderly patients. The side-effect of drowsiness may be reduced by giving a single daily dose at night.

amoxycillin A wide-range orally active penicillin very similar to ampicillin, but absorption is less influenced by food. It is active against a wide range of organisms and is used in the treatment of respiratory, urinary and soft tissue infections, and also in typhoid fever. *Dose:* 750mg–1.5g daily. In severe infections doses up to 4g daily by intravenous infusion. In simple, acute, urinary infections 2 doses of 3g with 12 hours between doses. In the prophylaxis of bacterial endocarditis 1 or 2 doses of 3g. The activity against penicillinase-producing organisms is increased by the combined use of clavulanic acid.

†**amphetamine sulphate** A powerful central nervous system stimulant. It is now rarely prescribed because of the high risk of dependence. See dexamphetamine.

amphotericin An antifungal antibiotic, effective in systemic as well as superficial infections. *Dose:* for systemic use, 250μg/kg daily in 5% glucose solution by intravenous infusion and increased if tolerated to a maximum of 1mg/kg daily. Side-effects, often severe, are numerous and include vomiting, fever, cardio- and nephrotoxicity. For intestinal candidiasis, doses of 400–800mg daily are given orally. For superficial infections 3% ointment is applied locally.

ampicillin An acid-stable and orally active penicillin with a wide range of activity similar to tetracycline. It is inactivated by penicillinase-producing organisms and most staphylococci are now resistant to ampicillin. It is used in chronic bronchitis, ear infections, and infections of the biliary and urinary tracts. *Dose:* 1–2g orally or by intramuscular injection; in severe infections, up to 4g daily by intravenous infusion. In urinary infections, doses of 1.5g daily are given, but in gonorrhoea, a single dose of 2g with 1g of probenecid is often effective, although females may require repeated doses. Skin reactions are relatively common but the urticarial type is indicative of penicillin allergy, and requires a change of treatment. A macropapular rash is frequent with patients with infective mononucleosis and treatment with ampicillin should be discontinued.

Ampiclox A mixed product containing ampicillin and cloxacillin.

amsacrine A synthetic cytotoxic agent similar in action to doxorubicin but less cardiotoxic. *Dose:* in refractory myeloid leukaemia, 90mg/m^2 daily for 5 days by intravenous infusion. Subsequent doses at intervals of 2–4 weeks according to response. Strict control is essential as hypokalaemia with fatal arrhythmia has occurred. Side-effects include nausea, stomatitis, alopecia, myelosuppression and epileptiform seizures.

amylobarbitone A barbiturate of medium intensity. *Dose:* 100–200mg. Sodium derivative is more rapid in action, but the effect less prolonged; it has been given intravenously for the control of convulsions and in epilepsy.

anabolic steroids Compounds related to testosterone with similar protein-building properties but reduced virilizing effects. They have been used to stimulate protein synthesis after major surgery and in wasting disease, but the response is sometimes disappointing. They are sometimes used to relieve the itching of chronic biliary obstruction, but may exacerbate the associated jaundice. Some anabolic steroids have been used in high doses in aplastic anaemia, and as palliatives in breast cancer. Side-effects are oedema and jaundice, and hepatic impairment is a contra-indication. They should not be given to children as they may cause premature closing of the epiphyses. See nandrolone and oxymetholone.

ancrod An anticoagulant obtained from the venom of a Malayan viper. It alters fibrinogen so that it does not react with thrombin to form fibrin, and any fibrin formed by other factors in the blood is rapidly removed by plasmin. The lower fibrinogen levels reduce blood viscosity, and the long action of ancrod is of value in deep vein thrombosis, retinal vein occlusion, embolism, vascular surgery and prophylactically post-operatively. *Dose:* 2–3 units/kg by slow intravenous infusion, repeated at 12-hourly intervals according to the plasma fibrinogen concentration. Haemorrhage is a possible side-effect, and if it is severe, may require the intravenous injection of ancrod-antivenom.

aneurine hydrochloride See thiamine.

angiotensin converting enzyme inhibitors Drugs which inhibit the conversion of angiotensin I (secreted by the kidney) to angiotensin II (a powerful hypertensive) and thus, indirectly, lower blood pressure. Angiotensin converting enzyme inhibitors are used in the treatment of hypertension, especially in severe conditions that have not responded to other therapy, and also in congestive heart failure. Initial therapy requires care, as a marked first-dose fall in blood pressure may occur. The first dose is best given at night, with the patient in bed, and if possible any diuretic treatment should have been suspended for a few days. Renal function should be monitored during angiotensin converting enzyme inhibitor therapy, as these drugs may cause a progressive and sometimes severe renal impairment. See captopril, enalapril, fosinopril, lisinopril, perindopril and quinapril. See also page 194.

anistreplase A complex of streptokinase with human plasminogen, used to restore blood flow after myocardial infarction. It binds with the fibrin of blood clots, and is slowly metabolized to release the active fibrinolytic agent plasmin. It is given by slow intravenous injection as a single dose of 30 units, within 6 hrs of infarction. Side-effects include transient hypotension, nausea, flushing and allergic reactions.

antazoline A mild antihistamine, used with the vasoconstrictor naphazoline as a nasal spray to reduce local congestion in sinusitis and rhinitis, and as eye-drops in allergic conjunctivitis.

antibiotics Antibacterial substances which occur as by-products of the growth of certain moulds. The term now includes some synthetic derivatives. The first to be discovered was penicillin and it remains the drug of choice in the treatment of many infections due to Gram-positive organisms as it is highly effective against susceptible cocci and is of low toxicity. Some penicillin derivatives (amoxycillin, ampicillin and mezlocillin) have a wider range of activity; others (cloxacillin, flucloxacillin and methicillin) are effective against resistant staphylococci, and carbenicillin, azlocillin, carfecillin, piperacillin and ticarcillin are effective against *Pseudomonas aeruginosa*. Antibiotics with a more extensive range of action are represented by aureomycin, chloramphenicol, the tetracyclines, and the cephalosporins. The aminoglycoside antibiotics represent antibiotics used mainly in infections due to Gram-negative organisms, but are more toxic than the penicillins or related drugs. Rifampicin is an antibiotic used mainly in tuberculosis. Broad-spectrum antibiotics should not be given for more than 5–10 days, to prevent disturbance of normal bacterial flora in the gut leading to overgrowth of fungal organisms such as candida.

Certain antibiotics, including neomycin and bacitracin, are too toxic for systemic use but may be useful in the treatment of infected skin conditions.

A few antibiotics such as actinomycin, bleomycin, doxorubicin, mitomycin and aclarubicin have cytotoxic properties. Others, such as griseofulvin, have only an antifungal action.

anticholinergic agents Drugs like atropine that inhibit the activity of the neurotransmitter acetylcholine. They are used as smooth muscle relaxants, as inhibitors of gastric secretion, and to reduce the excessive cholinergic activity associated with Parkinson's disease. By their nature, they have side-effects such as dryness of the mouth, blurred vision, and are contra-indicated in glaucoma. See page 210.

anticoagulants Blood clots consisting mainly of fibrin may form in the venous circulation, and heparin, ancrod and warfarin are used as anticoagulants in deep vein thrombosis. Heparin is also used prophylactically against post-operative thrombosis and during renal dialysis, and in low doses to reduce the risks of pulmonary embolism.

anticonvulsants Those drugs, also known as anti-epileptics, used to control the convulsions of epilepsy. The main types of convulsions or seizures are *grand mal* and *petit mal* (absence seizures) but atypical and myoclonic seizures may also occur. Some drugs are effective in most types of seizure, others are more selective, but in all cases dosage must be adjusted to need and response. Any change of treatment requires care with overlapping doses to avoid relapse. Paradoxically, young children may require relatively high doses. See page 192.

antidepressants The drugs used in the treatment of depression fall into two main groups, the so-called tricyclic antidepressants and the monoamine oxidase inhibitors. (Unrelated drugs include lithium carbonate, used only for the prophylaxis and treatment of manic depressive illness.) The tricyclic group, which now includes some tetracyclic and other compounds with a similar action, appear to act by blocking the neuronal uptake of central transmitters such as noradrenaline and serotonin. They are more widely used than the monoamine oxidase inhibitors because they are more generally effective, and react less extensively with other drugs and certain foods. The tricyclic drugs are widely used in endogenous depression, particularly when sleep disturbances are present, but the onset of action is slow, and improvement may not commence until after 2–4 weeks of treatment. Extended therapy is usually required to avoid the risk of a relapse. Some tricyclic antidepressants, such as amitriptyline, have a sedative action of value when anxiety is a complicating factor, whereas a less sedating drug such as imipramine may be useful in patients exhibiting apathy and withdrawal. Some of the side-effects, such as dryness of the mouth, are linked with their anticholinergic activity, but tolerance may develop with continued treatment. They also influence the cardiovascular system and may cause arrhythmias, tachycardia and hypotension, and may interfere with the action of some antihypertensive drugs, although the response to beta-blocking agents is unaffected. Care is necessary in cardiac disease, and with the elderly, initial doses should be low. The use of tricyclic antidepressants in epileptic patients may result in a lowering of the convulsive threshold. See page 185.

antidiabetic agents *Diabetes mellitus* is a deficiency disease due to a lack of insulin, and is characterized by an excessive level of glucose in the blood and urine. Treatment is either replacement therapy with daily injection of insulin, or orally by hypoglycaemic agents such as chlorpropamide. Such agents act by stimulating insulin secretion and release by the beta-cells of the pancreas, and are ineffective in the absence of such cells. See page 187.

anti-D(Rh_0)immunoglobulin Immunoglobulin is given to a rhesus-negative mother to prevent her forming antibodies against fetal rhesus-positive cells which may pass into the maternal circulation during childbirth or abortion and which, in a later pregnancy, could cause haemolytic disease. *Dose:* 500 units i.m. within 60–72 hrs of delivery or abortion. It is of no value if given after anti-D antibodies have been formed. The immunoglobulin has also been given after the transfusion of rhesus-incompatible blood.

antiemetics Nausea and vomiting may be due to several causes, including stimulation of the chemoreceptor trigger zone in the reticular formation of the brain. Many antiemetics have some degree of central activity, and in some cases their action may be mediated by blocking the effects of dopamine on the trigger zone. Effective drugs include some antihistamines, some phenothiazine-based tranquillizers such as prochlorperazine, whereas the alkaloid hyoscine is widely used in travel sickness. Others, such as domperidone, metoclopramide, nabilone and ondansetron, are of value in the control of the severe nausea and vomiting induced by cytotoxic drugs. The use of antiemetics in early pregnancy requires great care, and is seldom essential. See page 208.

antihistamines Drugs such as promethazine, of value in conditions associated with the release of histamine from mast cells, such as hayfever, rhinitis, urticaria, pruritus, and insect bites and stings. They are also useful in drug allergies. Some antihistamines have anti-emetic properties, and are useful in travel sickness. Although all antihistamines have the same basic action, the degree and duration of response and the severity of side-effects may vary. Some antihistamines pass easily into the central nervous system and are more likely to cause drowsiness. Others may have reduced anticholinergic properties, and cause less dryness of the mouth and blurring of vision. Care is necessary in epilepsy, glaucoma, hepatic disease or prostatic enlargement. See page 172.

antihypertensive agents See page 199.

anti-inflammatory agents See non-steroidal anti-inflammatory drugs and page 214.

antilymphocyte immunoglobulin An immunoglobulin obtained from immunized horses used as an immunosuppressive agent in transplant surgery to reduce the risk of rejection, and to supplement other immunosuppressive therapy. *Dose:* after a test-dose for possible sensitivity, 20–30mg/kg daily may be given by intravenous infusion for 3 weeks, followed by lower doses as required. Fever is a side-effect, and thrombophlebitis at the injection site may occur.

antimetabolites Cytotoxic drugs that appear to act by combining irreversibly with cell enzymes, and so prevent cell division. Methotrexate and mercaptopurine are examples.

antimuscarinic agents. See anticholinergic agents and page 210.

antineoplastic agents. Anti-cancer drugs. See page 180.

antitetanus immunoglobulin Human antitetanus immunoglobulin obtained from pooled plasma is used in injured patients who have not previously been immunized, and when tetanus is a definite risk. *Dose:* 250 units i.m. A course of tetanus vaccine should also be commenced.

antitubercular agents. See rifampicin.

apomorphine A morphine derivative formerly used by injection as a powerful emetic, but is now considered to be too toxic.

aprotinon An inhibitor of the proteolytic enzyme plasmin, obtained from bovine lung tissue. It is used in the severe haemorrhage due to hyperplasminaemia. *Dose:* 500 000–1 000 000 units by intravenous infusion.

arachis oil Groundnut or peanut oil. It has emollient properties, and is used in dermatology and pruritus as oily calamine lotion. Arachis oil enema is used to soften impacted faeces.

argipressin A synthetic form of vasopressin.

artificial tears Some chronic, sore eye conditions may occur in rheumatoid arthritis, and may be due to tear deficiency. Solutions of hypromellose, sometimes referred to as 'artificial tears', are useful as a bland lubricant to replace the tear deficiency.

ascorbic acid (vitamin C) Present in many citrus fruits. Deficiency is not uncommon in the elderly receiving inadequate diets. Severe deficiency causes scurvy, once the bane of seafarers. *Dose:* for prophylaxis 25–75mg daily; therapeutic dose 200–500mg daily. Doses of 4g daily are given for acidification of the urine. Claims that vitamin C prevents colds are unproven.

asparaginase Crisantaspase.

aspirin Acetylsalicylic acid. Widely used as a mild analgesic and anti-inflammatory agent, often in association with other drugs such as paracetamol and codeine. *Dose:* 300mg–1g but, in acute rheumatoid conditions, doses of 4–8g daily have been given. Long-term treatment with small doses (75mg) is given for the prophylaxis of cardiovascular disease. Side-effects include gastric irritation with some blood loss, hyperventilation, and tinnitus, with the risk of deafness, may occur with high doses. Aspirin may cause bronchospasm in asthmatic and other sensitive patients. As aspirin is now thought to be associated with Reye's syndrome, the drug should not be given to children under 12 years of age unless specifically indicated. Aspirin may increase the effects of certain hypoglycaemic and anticoagulant drugs. The anti-inflammatory action has been ascribed to the inhibition of prostaglandin synthesis.

astemizole An antihistamine with an extended action and reduced sedative effects. *Dose:* 10mg once daily before food. Larger doses up to 30mg daily may be given initially for a few days, but subsequently the 10mg daily dose *must not* be exceeded. Prolonged dosage in excess may cause cardiotoxic side-effects such as ventricular tachycardia.

atenolol A long-acting beta-adrenoceptor blocking agent of the propranolol type, but with a more cardioselective action. Used mainly in hypertension and angina. *Dose:* 50–100mg daily. Also given by slow intravenous injection in arrhythmias in doses up to 10mg. The side-effects are similar to propranolol, although atenolol may cause fewer sleep disturbances. See page 199.

atracurium A non-depolarizing muscle relaxant of the tubocurarine type, but causing less histamine release. *Dose:* 300–600μg/kg intravenously initially followed by doses of 100–200μg/kg at intervals as required. Its action can be reversed, if necessary, with neostigmine. Aminoglycoside antibiotics may increase the response and require an adjustment of dose.

atropine An alkaloid with anticholinergic properties obtained from belladonna, hyoscyamus and other plants, with powerful antispasmodic and mydriatic actions. It is often given in doses of 300–600μg by injection with morphine for pre-operative sedation and to reduce bronchial secretion, and is also of value in gastrointestinal smooth muscle spasm. *Dose:* 0.25–2mg daily. It is used as eye-drops (1%) to dilate the pupil, but such use in the elderly requires care, as the action may last as long as 7 days, and may precipitate glaucoma. It is also used with neostigmine in doses of 600μg–1.2mg to reverse the action of the tubocurarine-type muscle-relaxants. Side-effects include dryness of the mouth, disturbed vision, and bradycardia followed by tachycardia. Care is necessary in prostatic enlargement and urinary disturbances, and glaucoma is a contra-indication.

Augmentin See co-amoxiclav.

auranofin An orally active gold compound used in the treatment of active rheumatoid arthritis not relieved by non-steroidal anti-inflammatory drugs (NSAIDs). *Dose:* 6mg daily, increased if necessary after 6 months to 9mg daily. It should be withdrawn if the response is inadequate after nine months. Side-effects are nausea and diarrhoea. See sodium aurothiomalate for the systemic side-effects of gold therapy.

Avomine Derivative of promethazine used in travel sickness, nausea and vomiting. *Dose:* 25–150mg daily.

azapropazone A non-steroidal anti-inflammatory agent with actions and uses similar to those of naproxen. *Dose:* 1.2g daily, but in acute gout an initial, divided, dose of 2.4g is given. Side-effects include rash and occasional photosensitivity, and care is necessary in peptic ulcer. Azapropazone may potentiate the action of warfarin and phenytoin, and require an adjustment of dose.

azatadine An antihistamine with the actions and uses of promethazine, *Dose:* 1mg twice daily.

azathioprine An immunosuppressive agent used to inhibit rejection after organ transplant surgery. Also of value in chronic hepatitis, systemic lupus erythematosus, pemphigus and other conditions resistant to corticosteroid therapy. *Dose:* 1–5mg/kg daily, but dose and duration vary according to need and response. Side-effects include depression of bone marrow function, gastrointestinal disturbances, hepatotoxicity and rash. Severe secondary infections may occur as a result of the immunosuppression, and the use of the drug requires close control.

azidothymidine See zidovudine.

azithromycin A macrolide antibiotic with a longer action than erythromycin or clarithromycin, used chiefly in respiratory tract infections. *Dose:* 500mg daily for 3 days, 1 hour before or 2 hours after food or antacids. Side-effects include nausea, abdominal discomfort and diarrhoea.

azlocillin A broad-spectrum antibiotic with exceptional activity against *Pseudomonas*. Of value in respiratory and urinary infections, and in septicaemia. It is inactivated by penicillinase-producing organisms, but combined use with a penicillin of the cloxacillin-type may increase the activity. *Dose:* in life-threatening infections, 5g by intravenous infusion 8-hrly. Doses of 2g 8-hrly may be given in less severe infections. In patients with impaired renal function, doses should be given 12-hrly. Allergy to penicillins or cephalosporins is a contra-indication.

AZT See zidovudine.

aztreonam An antibiotic that is exceptional in being resistant to breakdown by beta-lactamases, yet it has a selective action against Gram-negative aerobes, with little effect on Gram-positive bacteria or bowel organisms. It is given in urinary, respiratory, bone and other infections caused by susceptible bacteria, and may be given with other antibiotics in mixed infections or pending susceptibility tests. When given in association with an aminoglycoside, the activity of aztreonam against *Pseudomonas aeruginosa* may be increased. *Dose:* 4g daily by intramuscular injection and up to 8g daily intravenously in severe infections. Reduced doses are indicated in renal impairment. Although aztreonam has some aminoglycoside-like activity, it is less liable to cause nephro- or ototoxicity. Side-effects are skin reactions, nausea, jaundice and malaise. Aztreonam may increase prothrombin times.

B

BIPP A mixture of bismuth subnitrate, iodoform, and liquid paraffin, used as an antiseptic dressing, applied on gauze.

bacampicillin A derivative of ampicillin, which is rapidly hydrolysed after absorption to give high peak blood levels of ampicillin. *Dose:* 1.2 – 2.4g daily. In gonorrhoea, 1.6g as a single dose, with 1g of probenecid to prolong the action. The side-effects are those of ampicillin.

bacitracin An antibiotic used by local application. It is too toxic for systemic use.

baclofen A muscle relaxant that acts on the spinal end of some motor neurones. Useful in multiple sclerosis and muscle spasms caused by spinal lesions. *Dose:* 15mg daily initially gradually increased, as required, up to a maximum of 100mg daily. Side-effects include nausea, fatigue and hypotension. Care is necessary in epilepsy and psychiatric disorders.

BAL See dimercaprol.

†**barbiturates** A group of hypnotic drugs exemplified by butobarbitone. Once widely used, but their value has declined sharply as safer drugs such as nitrazepam have been introduced.

barium sulphate A very insoluble powder, given orally or rectally as an aqueous suspension as contrast agent for X-ray examination of the alimentary system. *Note: soluble* salts of barium are very poisonous.

BCG vaccine A preparation of the Calmette-Guérin strain of

Mycobacterium tuberculosis. It is used for active immunization against tuberculosis, particularly for individuals likely to be exposed to infection. *Dose:* 0.1mL by intradermal injection. A product obtained from an isoniazid-resistant strain of the organism is also used for the immunization of individuals receiving prophylactic treatment with isoniazid.

beclomethasone A potent corticosteroid used in the control of asthma and bronchospasm not responding to other drugs. *Dose:* by oral aerosol inhalation, 100μg (two puffs) repeated up to four times a day according to need and response. *Dose:* by powder inhalation 800μg daily. Hoarseness may develop as a side-effect, and oral candidiasis may occur with high doses. Beclomethasone is also used as a cream or ointment (0.025%) in severe inflammatory skin conditions not responding to less potent corticosteroids.

belladonna The deadly nightshade (*Atropa belladonna*). The principal constituent is atropine.

bendrofluazide A widely used diuretic of the thiazide group, with a powerful and prolonged action. It is used in congestive heart failure, oedema and mild hypertension. In more severe hypertension it is given together with other drugs to increase the overall response. *Dose:* 2.5–10mg daily. It causes some loss of potassium, so potassium supplements are required if treatment is prolonged. Side-effects include rash and thrombocytopenia. Renal failure is a contra-indication. See page 194.

benorylate A compound of aspirin and paracetamol, with the general properties of both drugs, but generally better tolerated than aspirin. Used in arthritic conditions and for the relief of painful musculoskeletal disorders. *Dose:* 3–6g daily. Like aspirin, it may cause gastrointestinal disturbances and increase the action of oral anticoagulants.

benperidol A tranquillizer of the haloperidol type with similar side-effects, but used to control antisocial sexual behaviour in adults. *Dose:* 0.25–1.5mg daily.

benserazide An enzyme inhibitor used with levodopa in parkinsonism. It inhibits the breakdown of levodopa to dopamine, and so permits a reduction in dose and a smoother response. Some of the side-effects of levodopa, such as nausea and vomiting, may also be reduced, although the incidence of involuntary movements may increase. *Dose:* 12.5mg with 50mg of levodopa.

benzalkonium chloride A detergent with antiseptic properties present in various skin preparations. It is also used as a preservative in eye-drops.

benzathine penicillin A long-acting penicillin compound; present in Penidural.

benzhexol hydrochloride A spasmolytic drug used mainly to relieve the tremor and rigidity of parkinsonism. *Dose:* 1mg initially, slowly increased to 5–15mg daily according to need. Side-effects include mouth dryness, dizziness and blurred vision. Care is necessary with high doses as some psychiatric disturbances may occur and warrant withdrawal of the drug, but abrupt discontinuance of treatment should be avoided. Benzhexol should be used with care in cases of glaucoma, hepatic and cardiac disease or urinary disturbances.

benzocaine A local anaesthetic for topical application. Used as lozenges (100mg) for painful oral conditions; ointment (5–10%); suppositories 200mg.

benzodiazepines A widely used group of drugs with a powerful action on the central nervous system. They appear to have a selective action on certain serotonin receptors. The type of action varies within the group, and they may be used as sedatives, hypnotics, anxiolytics, anticonvulsants or muscle relaxants. As hypnotics they have virtually replaced the barbiturates, as they have a wide margin of safety and are less dangerous in overdose. Prolonged use should be avoided as dependence remains a possibility. The withdrawal of treatment with benzodiazepines should be gradual, as otherwise confusion, convulsions and toxic psychoses may occur. Nitrazepam has a relatively long action as a hypnotic, whereas flunitrazepam has a shorter action. Diazepam is the preferred drug for controlling the spasms of tetanus. Hypnotic benzodiazepines include flunitrazepam, flurazepam, loprazolam, lormetazepam, nitrazepam, temazepam and triazolam. Those used as anxiolytics are alprazolam, bromazepam, chlordiazepoxide, clobazam, clorazepate, diazepam, ketazolam, lorazepam, medazepam, oxazepam and pramazepam. Most of these diazepines are referred to briefly under the above names. See also pages 176 and 202.

benzoic acid It has fungistatic properties similar to salicylic acid, and has been used as Whitfield's ointment (Compound Benzoic Acid Ointment) for the treatment of ringworm.

benzoin A balsamic resin used mainly as Compound Tincture of Benzoin for pressure sores and stoma care.

benzoyl peroxide An antifungal agent used locally for superficial fungal infections. It is also used, together with sulphur, as a cream or gel for acne.

benzthiazide A thiazide diuretic present with triamterene in Dytide.

benztropine An anticholinergic drug, used to relieve the rigidity, tremor and salivation of Parkinson's disease. It also has some sedative action, and in some cases may be preferred to benzhexol. Like benzhexol, it is sometimes useful in the control of drug-induced extrapyramidal symptoms. *Dose:* 0.5–6mg daily. In severe conditions, it may be given by injection of 1–2mg, repeated according to response. The side-effects are those of the anticholinergic drugs generally.

benzydamine A mild analgesic used as a mouthwash (0.15%) for painful conditions of the mouth and throat, and as a cream (3%) for musculo-skeletal pain.

benzyl benzoate A clear liquid with an aromatic odour. It is used as an emulsion in the treatment of scabies by two applications to the whole of the body except the head.

benzyl penicillin See penicillin.

bephenium An anthelmintic effective against hookworm and roundworm. *Dose:* 2.5g on an empty stomach, with a second dose after 1 or 2 days. Nausea, diarrhoea, dizziness and headache are occasional side-effects.

beta-adrenoceptor blocking agents Adrenaline and related catecholamines are released into the circulation during exercise and stress, and stimulate cardiac output by acting on the beta-adrenoceptor sites in the heart. When such stimulation is excessive the increased oxygen demand of the heart may cause myocardial insufficiency and angina. Drugs such as propranolol block these receptor sites and so indirectly reduce cardiac stimulation, and are of value in the control of angina, cardiac arrhythmias and hypertension. Some blocking agents also act on other receptor sites and may cause bronchospasm by releasing histamine. Newer drugs, represented by acebutolol and metoprolol, are more cardioselective, and others such as sotalol are of more value in hypertension. Some of these blocking agents, such as atenolol, are less likely to reach the central nervous system, and so may cause fewer sleep disturbances. By their nature and depressant action on the myocardium, care is necessary when giving beta-blockers in cardiac failure, heart block and bradycardia. See pages 199 and 206.

betahistine A vasodilator with some of the properties of histamine. Used to reduce the vertigo of Ménière's disease. Should be used with care in asthmatics and in peptic ulcer. *Dose:* 16–48mg daily.

betamethasone A synthetic corticosteroid characterized by the low dose, increased anti-inflammatory action, and reduced side-effects. It has virtually no salt-retaining properties, and causes little increase in the urinary excretion of potassium. It is indicated in all inflammatory, allergic and other conditions requiring corticosteroid therapy – with the exception of Addison's disease and after adrenalectomy when a salt-retaining steroid is required. *Dose:* 0.5–5mg daily; in cerebral oedema, 5–20mg by intramuscular or intravenous injection. In asthmatic states, oral aerosol inhalation of 800μg (eight puffs) daily; for inflammatory conditions of the eye, ear and nose, a 0.1% solution used locally.

betaxolol A beta-adrenoceptor blocking agent of the propranolol type, with similar properties and side-effects, but with a more cardio-selective action. It is used mainly in the treatment of hypertension. *Dose:* 20mg once daily. Betaxolol is also used as eye-drops (0.5%) in ocular hypertension and glaucoma.

bethanechol A parasympathomimetic agent used in paralytic ileus and post-operative urinary retention. *Dose:* 30–120mg daily before food. Side-effects are nausea, bradycardia and colic. Care is necessary in asthma and cardiovascular disease.

bethanidine A blocking agent that has an antihypertensive action by inhibiting the release of noradrenaline from post-ganglionic adrenergic nerve endings. It is useful in resistant hypertension, and when other agents are not well tolerated, and is usually given in association with a thiazide diuretic or a beta blocker. *Dose:* 20–200mg daily. Postural hypotension, nasal congestion and diarrhoea are side-effects.

bezafibrate A plasma-lipid regulating agent with an action similar to clofibrate, and used in the treatment of hyperlipidaemia not responding to diet. *Dose:* 600mg daily with food. Contra-indicated in renal or hepatic dysfunction. May potentiate oral anticoagulants. Side-effects are nausea, pruritus and urticaria. See page 197.

biperiden An antispasmodic and parasympatholytic drug

used chiefly to control the rigidity and excessive salivation of parkinsonism. It has less effect on tremor. *Dose:* 2mg daily initially, increased, as required, up to 6mg or more daily. If necessary it may be given by intramuscular or slow intravenous injection in doses of 5–20mg daily. Side-effects include dizziness, blurred vision and drowsiness.

bisacodyl A synthetic laxative that exerts its action by a direct stimulating effect on the nerve endings of the colon. *Dose:* 10mg orally, or as a suppository. Abdominal cramp is an occasional side-effect. It should not be used in intestinal obstruction.

bismuth chelate A potassium-bismuth-citrate complex used to promote the healing of peptic ulcers, mainly by a protective action. *Dose:* 480mg daily for 28 days, repeated if necessary at monthly intervals. Not to be given with food. It may blacken the faeces. See page 212.

bismuth subgallate A yellow insoluble powder with astringent properties. Used as dusting powder, and as suppositories for rectal conditions.

bisoprolol A beta-blocking agent with the actions, uses and side-effects of propranolol. It is given in hypertension and angina in doses of 5–20mg daily.

bleomycin A cytotoxic antibiotic, exceptional in causing little if any disturbance of bone marrow activity. Used mainly in skin tumours, lymphomas, and mycosis fungoides. *Dose:* 15–30mg twice-weekly by intramuscular or intravenous injection up to a total dose of 500mg. The onset of stomatitis is an indication of the maximum tolerated dose. Pigmentation of the skin may occur, but a severe dose-related, delayed reaction is pulmonary fibrosis, requiring immediate withdrawal of the drug. There is a risk of respiratory failure during general anaesthesia associated with a high oxygen intake.

boric acid, boracic acid Mild antiseptic. Should not be applied to large, raw areas owing to risk of absorption in toxic amounts. It is also used in the preparation of eusol.

bretylium An antihypertensive agent, now used only in the control of resistant ventricular arrhythmias. *Dose:* 5mg/kg, i.m., 6–8-hrly. It may also be given by slow intravenous injection in doses of 5–10mg/kg, repeated as required. Side-effects include nausea, vomiting and severe hypotension.

brilliant green An antiseptic dye formerly used as a paint (0.5%) with crystal violet for skin preparation.

bromazepam A benzodiazepine used mainly in the short-term treatment of anxiety. *Dose:* 9–18mg daily. Contra-indicated in respiratory depression and phobic states.

bromocriptine An inhibitor of the release of prolactin from the pituitary gland. It is used to prevent or suppress lactation when other measures have failed. *Dose:* 2.5mg daily initially for a few days, then twice daily for 14 days. It also stimulates dopamine receptors in the brain, and it is used in parkinsonism, mainly in patients unable to tolerate levodopa, to stimulate any surviving dopamine receptors. *Dose:* 1.25mg at night initially, with food, slowly increased according to response up to 40mg. The use of the drug requires care, as it has many side-effects, including early hypotensive reactions. See page 210. Bromocriptine is also used in some conditions of pituitary dysfunction such as acromegaly.

brompheniramine An antihistamine similar to promethazine, but with a shorter action and reduced side-effects. It also has some anti-tussive properties. *Dose:* 12–32mg daily.

budesonide A steroid similar to beclomethasone, and used by oral aerosol inhalation in chronic airway obstruction and other asthmatic conditions. *Dose:* 200–800μg (1–4 puffs) according to need.

bufexamac An analgesic and anti-inflammatory agent that has been used orally for rheumatic conditions. It is now used mainly as a 5% cream for the treatment of mildly inflamed skin conditions.

bumetanide A rapidly acting loop diuretic similar to frusemide, with comparable actions, uses and side-effects. *Dose:* 1–5mg daily. Much larger doses may be needed when renal function is impaired. In acute pulmonary and cardiac oedema, 1–2mg may be given intravenously.

bupivacaine A local anaesthetic related to lignocaine but characterized by its increased potency and long duration of action which may be up to 8 hrs when used for nerve blocks. It is also of value in continuous epidural analgesia. It is used as a 0.25% to 0.5% solution in doses according to requirements with or without adrenaline. The side-effects are those of lignocaine, but it may cause more severe myocardial depression.

buprenorphine A powerful analgesic, related to morphine, but less likely to cause dependence. Valuable in pain of terminal cancer, after operation or myocardial infarction. *Dose:* 200–400μg 6–8-hrly as sublingual tablets, or 300–600μg by intramuscular or slow intravenous injection at intervals of 6–8 hrs according to need. Side-effects include drowsiness, nausea and dizziness. Naloxone is a partial antagonist.

buserelin A synthetic gonadotrophin-releasing hormone that indirectly depresses the level of serum testosterone. It is used in the treatment of testosterone-sensitive prostatic carcinoma. *Dose:* 500μg by subcutaneous injection 8-hrly for 7 days, followed by intranasal maintenance doses of 100μg 6 times a day. Patients should be warned that an increase in pain may occur initially. Side-effects are hot flushes and loss of libido.

buspirone A new drug for the treatment of anxiety. It may act like the benzodiazepines on serotonin receptors in the brain, but the full response may take 1–2 weeks. *Dose:* 10–15mg daily initially, slowly increased as required up to a maximum of 45mg daily. Side-effects are nausea, dizziness and drowsiness. Benzodiazepines must be withdrawn slowly before transfer to buspirone. See page 176.

busulphan A cytotoxic compound used in the palliative treatment of chronic myeloid leukaemia. Close haematological control is essential during treatment as remission of symptoms may not be complete for some weeks and overdose may cause irreversible myelodepression. *Dose:* 0.5–4mg daily. Side-effects include pigmentation of the skin.

†**butobarbitone** A barbiturate of medium intensity and rapidity of onset. *Dose:* 60–200mg.

butriptyline An antidepressant with the actions, uses and side-effects of amitriptyline, but with a reduced sedative action. *Dose:* 75–150mg daily.

C

CCNU Lomustine.

cade oil An old treatment for psoriasis and some forms of eczema. Used as ointment and shampoo, and as medicated soap for seborrhoea.

cadexomer iodine A modified starch powder containing 0.9% of iodine in a slow release form. It is used as an antiseptic application for venous ulcers and pressure sores. It should not be used during pregnancy or lactation, during thyroid investigations or in patients sensitive to iodine.

caffeine The central nervous system stimulant present in tea and coffee. It is used with paracetamol and other mild analgesics. *Dose:* 100–300mg. Caffeine sodium benzoate is a soluble compound used by injection as a cardiac and respiratory stimulant. *Dose:* 0.3–1g.

calamine Zinc carbonate. It has a mild astringent and soothing action when applied to the skin, and is widely used as Calamine Lotion for skin irritation and as Oily Calamine Lotion in eczema.

calciferol (vitamin D_2) The form of vitamin D used in the prophylaxis and treatment of deficiency states such as rickets in children and osteomalacia in adults, and in other bone disorders. *Dose:* prophylactic 800 units daily; therapeutic 5000–50 000 units daily. In resistant rickets and parathyroid deficiency, higher doses may be required, but such therapy requires care, as hypercalcaemia and irreversible renal damage may occur. See also alfacalcidol and calcitriol.

calcipotriol Some analogues of vitamin D have certain inhibitory effects on cell growth. Calcipotriol is a new derivative with little effect on calcium metabolism, but an increased action against the proliferation of keratinocytes. It is used as a 0.005% ointment in the treatment of psoriasis vulgaris, and is applied to the plaques twice daily. A course of treatment should not exceed 5 weeks.

calcitonin Pork-derived calcitonin is a hormone that has an action similar to that of the parathyroid gland in regulating blood calcium levels. It is used in the hypercalcaemia associated with malignancy, and in osteoporosis. It is also of value in Paget's disease of bone, in which it relieves bone pain and reduces the neurological symptoms. *Dose:* 10–160 units daily by subcutaneous or intramuscular injection according to need and response. In Paget's disease, prolonged treatment for some months may be required. Side-effects are nausea, flushing and paraesthesia, and local reactions may also occur. See salcatonin.

calcitriol The metabolite formed in the kidney from calciferol. It is the most powerful and rapidly acting metabolite with vitamin D activity. It is of value in chronic renal deficiency states when the normal metabolism of calcium and phosphorus is impaired, as in renal osteodystrophy. *Dose:* 1–2μg daily under biochemical control. Side-effects, such as hypercalcaemia and hypercalciuria, are usually reversible on withdrawing the drug.

calcium-channel blocking agents

The movement of calcium ions through the calcium channels of the myocardium plays an essential role in cardiac activity. The inhibition of such movement by channel-blocking agents reduces myocardial contractility and lowers the tone of the cardiovascular system. Such a reduction is of value in angina, hypertension and cardiac arrhythmias, and can be obtained by the use of calcium-channel blocking agents such as diltiazem, felodipine, isradipine, nicardipine, nifedipine, nimidopine and verapamil. These compounds exhibit certain differences in therapeutic applications, and their use requires care. Nifedipine and verapamil have been used in the prophylactic treatment of migraine. Their side-effects include nausea, oedema, rash and bradycardia.

calcium carbonate Chalk.

calcium chloride The calcium salt present in various intravenous electrolyte solutions.

calcium folinate See folinic acid.

calcium gluconate A soluble and well-tolerated calcium salt used in many conditions associated with calcium deficiency such as rickets, coeliac disease, and parathyroid deficiency; also during pregnancy and lactation often in association with vitamin D. Calcium gluconate is also given in chilblains, urticaria and allergic reactions. It is usually given in doses of 0.5–2g, but in hypocalcaemic tetany it is given by slow intravenous injection in doses of 10ml of a 10% solution, with laboratory control of the blood calcium levels. Calcium gluconate is also given intravenously in the early treatment of toxic hyperkalaemia.

calcium lactate The calcium salt most commonly given orally in mild deficiency states. *Dose:* 1–5g.

Calcium Resonium An ion-exchange resin that takes up potassium in exchange for calcium. Used in hyperkalaemia associated with anuria and haemodialysis. Should be used only when potassium and calcium serum levels are under biochemical control. *Dose:* 15–30g three or four times a day. In children, 0.5–1g/kg daily. It is sometimes given as a retention enema.

camphor A white crystalline substance with an aromatic odour. It is used externally as a solution in arachis oil (camphorated oil), as a rubifacient and mild analgesic in fibrositis and similar conditions. Poisoning, with nausea and convulsions, has occurred when the solution has been swallowed, and the use of camphorated oil is now discouraged.

canrenoate A steroid-derived aldosterone antagonist with the actions and uses of spironolactone. It is given in oedema by slow intravenous injection or infusion in doses of 200–400mg daily. Nausea and vomiting are high-dose side-effects.

capreomycin An antibiotic of value in resistant tuberculosis or when other drugs are not tolerated. *Dose:* 1g daily by intramuscular injection. It may cause tinnitus, deafness, renal damage and allergic reactions.

captopril An inhibitor of the angiotensin converting enzyme. It is used in the treatment of hypertension, including that resistant to other therapy, but care is necessary as the initial dose may cause marked hypotension, and so is best taken in bed. It is often given with a thiazide diuretic to improve the response, and with a beta-blocker to maintain the effect. *Dose:* 25mg initially slowly increased, as required, up to 450mg daily. Similar doses are given in heart failure. Side-effects include proteinuria, neutropenia, agranulocytosis, rash and loss of taste. See ACE inhibitors.

carbachol A parasympathomimetic agent used orally and by injection in the treatment of post-operative atony and retention of urine, and occasionally as eye-drops (3%) in the treatment of glaucoma. *Dose:* 2–4mg orally, 250μg by subcutaneous injection. Side-effects include nausea, bradycardia and colic.

carbamazepine An anticonvulsant effective in all types of epilepsy except petit mal (absence seizures). It is also of value in trigeminal neuralgia and is given prophylactically in manic-depressive states. *Dose:* 200–400mg daily initially, slowly increased up to 1.8g daily if required. Carbamazepine has some anti-diuretic properties, and has been used in diabetes insipidus. Side-effects include dizziness, gastrointestinal disturbances, and an erythematous rash. See page 192.

carbaryl An insecticide used as a lotion and shampoo in pediculosis.

carbenicillin A derivative of penicillin of lower potency but a wider range of activity. Of value in systemic and urinary infections due to *Pseudomonas aeruginosa*, *Proteus*, and mixed infections although ticarcillin is more potent, and is often preferred. *Dose:* In severe systemic infections, 20–30g daily by rapid intravenous infusion; for urinary infections, 1–2g 6-hourly i.m. Smaller doses should be given when the renal function is impaired. Carfenicillin is an orally active derivative.

carbenoxolone A derivative obtained from liquorice. It has some anti-inflammatory properties and is used in the treatment of gastric and duodenal ulcer, and locally for mouth ulcers. *Dose:* 300mg daily initially, and subsequently 150mg daily for some weeks. Side-effects include oedema and heartburn, and potassium supplements may be necessary to prevent hypokalaemia. Care is necessary in hepatic and renal dysfunction. See page 212.

carbidopa An enzyme inhibitor used with levodopa in parkinsonism. It prevents the breakdown of levodopa, thus permitting a larger amount to reach the brain.

carbimazole An antithyroid drug. It inhibits the formation of thyroxine and is valuable in the treatment of thyrotoxicosis and in preparation for thyroidectomy. *Dose:* 30–60mg daily initially; maintenance doses, 5–20mg daily. It is sometimes given together with thyroxine in the 'blockage-replacement' treatment of hyperthyroidism. Side-effects are nausea, rash and pruritus; alopecia and agranulocytosis have been reported.

carbocisteine A mucolytic agent used to reduce the production and viscosity of sputum in respiratory disorders. *Dose:* 1.5g daily.

carbolic acid Phenol, *q.v.*

carbon dioxide A colourless, non-inflammable gas. It has a stimulating effect on the respiratory centre, and a mixture of 5% of carbon dioxide in oxygen is used for respiratory depression. Solid carbon dioxide is used to destroy warts, naevi, etc.

carbonic anhydrase inhibitors These drugs, represented by acetazolamide and dichlorphenamide, have been used as diuretics as they inhibit the reabsorption of sodium and bicarbonate in the kidneys, and so produce an alkaline urine. Their use has declined as more effective diuretics have become available, but as they also reduce the formation of the aqueous humour and so bring about a reduction in the intra-ocular pressure, they are also used in the treatment of glaucoma.

carboplatin An analogue of cisplatin but with generally reduced side-effects, although the myelodepression may be more severe. It is used mainly in ovarian and small-cell lung cancer. *Dose:* 40mg/m^2 intravenously as a single dose, repeated after 4 weeks. Blood tests during treatment are essential. Severe renal impairment is a contra-indication.

carboprost A prostaglandin with a selective action on the myometrium, and used in the post-partum haemorrhage not responding to ergometrine. *Dose:* 250μg initially by deep intramuscular injection, with subsequent doses according to need up to a total of 12mg (not for intravenous injection). Care in asthma, epilepsy and hypertension. Nausea and vomiting are side-effects.

carfecillin An orally active derivative of carbenicillin, that is metabolized after absorption to yield low blood levels of the active drug. These low levels are inadequate for the treatment of systemic infections, but as the metabolite is excreted in an active form in the urine, carficillin is correspondingly useful in urinary infections due to *Pseudomonas* and *Proteus*. *Dose:* 1.5–3g daily. The side-effects are those of penicillin.

carisoprodol A muscle relaxant that reduces muscle tone by a central action. Useful in musculoskeletal disorders and muscle spasm. *Dose:* 1g daily, often with paracetamol. Drowsiness is a common side-effect.

carmustine A cytotoxic agent similar to lomustine. It is used mainly in brain tumours, multiple myeloma, and Hodgkin's disease, often in association with other drugs. *Dose:* 200mg/m^2 by slow intravenous injection, repeated at intervals of 6 weeks. Side-effects are nausea, vomiting and burning at the injection site. A delayed bone-marrow depression is often a dose-limiting factor.

carteolol A beta-adrenergic blocking agent used in the treatment of angina. *Dose:* 10–30mg daily. It is also used as eye-drops (0.1–0.2%) in glaucoma. Some systemic absorption may occur from eye-drops, and care is necessary in asthma and bradycardia.

cascara A mild purgative. *Dose:* dry extract 100–250mg, liquid extract and elixir, 2–5ml.

castor oil A mild purgative, often useful after food poisoning. *Dose:* 5–20ml. The oil has emollient properties and is used together with zinc ointment for pressure sores, and napkin rash.

catecholamines A term applied to the sympathomimetic drugs adrenaline, dopamine, noradrenaline, and related compounds, indicating that they are derivatives of catechol.

catechu A plant extract used with chalk in the treatment of diarrhoea. It is a constituent of Aromatic Chalk and Opium Mixture.

cefaclor An orally active cephalosporin antibiotic used mainly in urinary and respiratory infections. *Dose*: 750mg, or more, up to 4g daily, with reduced doses in renal impairment. Nausea and diarrhoea are side-effects, but an allergic reaction indicating sensitivity may require withdrawal of the drug.

cefadroxil An analogue of cephalexin. It is well absorbed orally and gives high blood levels. *Dose:* 1–2g, daily.

cefamandole Cephamandole.

cefixime A cephalosporin with the actions, uses and side-effects of the cephalosporins generally, but effective in single daily doses of 200–400mg.

cefotaxime A cephalosporin antibiotic with an increased activity against many Gram-negative organisms. *Dose:* 2g daily by injection, increased in severe infections up to 12g daily. A single dose of 1g is given in gonorrhoea. The side-effects are those of the cephalosporins generally.

cefoxitin A cephamycin antibiotic with a wide range of activity and an increased potency against Gram-negative bacteria. It is of value in many infections, and is also used in surgical prophylaxis. *Dose:* 3–12g daily by intramuscular or intravenous injection. Side-effects are those of the cephalosporins generally.

cefsulodin A semi-synthetic cephalosporin effective against *Pseudomonas aeruginosa*, including strains resistant to carbenicillin and gentamicin. It is excreted unchanged in the urine, and is of value in urinary, respiratory and soft-tissue infections. *Dose:* 1–4g daily by intramuscular or intravenous injection.

ceftazidime A cephalosporin antibiotic resistant to most beta-lactamases, and active against a wide range of Gram-positive and Gram-negative organisms, including *Pseudomonas aeruginosa*, although it is less active against *Staphylococcus aureus*. Valuable in both single and mixed infections. *Dose:* 1–6g daily by injection, reduced in cases of renal impairment. In pseudomonal lung infections associated with cystic fibrosis, 100–150mg/kg daily. Side-effects include abdominal disturbance and local reactions at the injection site.

ceftizoxime A broad-spectrum antibiotic with the general properties of the cephalosporins. Useful in a wide range of single or mixed infections, but less effective against *Staphylococcus aureus*. *Dose:* up to 8g daily by injection; in urinary infections 1–2g daily; in gonorrhoea a single intramuscular dose of 1g. Side-effects include pain at the injection site, nausea, and diarrhoea.

cefuroxime A cephalosporin antibiotic, often effective against some organisms resistant to penicillin, and with increased activity against *Haemophilus influenzae*. *Dose:* up to 6g daily by injection. For surgical prophylaxis and in gonorrhoea a single dose of 1.5g. Side-effects include nausea, diarrhoea, urticaria, rash and hypersensitivity reactions. An orally active form is cefuroxime-axetil. *Dose:* 500mg–1g daily.

celiprolol A selective β_1 receptor blocking agent, with some stimulating action on β_2 receptors. The former occur mainly in the heart, the latter in the bronchi and peripheral vessels. It is used in mild hypertension, as it has a vasodilatory and cardioselective action with reduced side-effects. *Dose:* 200mg daily, with water, before breakfast. Occasional side-effects are nausea, headache and dizziness.

cephalexin An orally active cephalosporin of value in infections of the respiratory and urinary tracts, and in naso-oral and soft-tissue infections, including those caused by sensitive *Staphylococci*. *Dose:* 1–2g daily, but lower doses are indicated in renal impairment. Cephalexin is usually well-tolerated, but some gastro-intestinal disturbances may occur.

cephalosporins A group of antibiotics with properties similar to those of the penicillins, but having a wider range of activity. Some are active orally, others may have to be given by injection. Cefotaxime, ceftazidime and ceftizoxime have an increased activity against Gram-negative bacteria, but are less potent against *Staphylococcus aureus* and Gram-positive organisms generally. Cefoxitin is active against bowel organisms, and cefsulidin is effective in pseudomonal infections. An indication of the dose-range is given in the table on page 267. The higher doses are given in severe infections; reduced doses should be given in renal impairment. The main side-effect of the cephalosporins is hypersensitivity, and cross-sensitivity to the penicillins is not uncommon. Sensitivity to one is likely to extend to all members of the group. The cephalosporins can affect blood-clotting mechanisms.

cephalothin One of the first cephalosporins, now largely replaced by more active derivatives. *Dose:* 4–12g daily by injection. It is inactive orally.

cephamandole A cephalosporin more resistant to inactivation by penicillinases. It is of value in serious infections resistant to other antibiotics.

Dose: 2–12g daily by intramuscular or intravenous injection.

cephamycins A small group of antibiotics closely related to the cephalosporins and having similar actions and uses. See cefoxitin.

cephazolin A cephalosporin with the general properties of the group. *Dose:* 2–12g daily by injection.

cephradine A cephalosporin active orally as well as by injection. *Dose:* 1–2g orally daily; in severe infections, 2–8g daily by injection.

cetirizine A new slower-acting antihistamine with reduced sedative effects, as it does not pass the blood-brain barrier to any extent. The anticholinergic side-effects are also reduced. *Dose:* 10mg at night.

cetrimide A detergent with some antiseptic properties. It is used chiefly in association with chlorhexidine.

chalk Also known as calcium carbonate, chalk has been used as an antacid, but it may cause some rebound acid secretion. It is now used chiefly as an adsorbent in diarrhoea, often together with astringents as in Aromatic Chalk and Opium Mixture.

charcoal Activated charcoal is a powerful adsorbent, and is used in the treatment of overdose or poisoning by many toxic drugs by preventing further absorption. *Dose:* 50g orally. It is also used in the charcoal haemoperfusion system to promote elimination from the circulation of some already absorbed poisons such as central depressants. Charcoal has also been used in small doses in the treatment of flatulence, and as a marker for the passage of faeces. *Dose:* 4–8g.

chenodeoxycholic acid A bile acid-derivative that has a solvent action on cholesterol-containing gallstones, and it is useful when surgical removal of the stones is contra-indicated. *Dose:* 1g once daily, but prolonged treatment is necessary, and should be continued for some weeks after the dissolution of the stones has been confirmed. Side-effects are diarrhoea and pruritus, and ursodeoxycholic acid, which has fewer side-effects is often preferred. Chenodeoxycholic acid is not suitable for the dissolution of radio-opaque gallstones.

chloral hydrate A water-soluble hypnotic with a rapid action that is useful in the treatment of insomnia in children and the elderly. *Dose:* 0.3–2g. It must be given well-diluted to reduce the gastric irritant side-effects, and is contra-indicated in gastritis, and severe renal, hepatic and cardiac disease. Chloral betaine (Welldorm) is a less irritant alternative.

chlorambucil An orally active cytotoxic drug used mainly in the treatment of lymphomas and chronic lymphocytic leukaemia. *Dose:* 100–200μg/kg daily for 4–8 weeks. It is sometimes used as an immunosuppressant in the treatment of rheumatoid arthritis in doses of 2.5–7.5mg daily. Chlorambucil is generally well tolerated, but bone marrow depression may occur, and haematological control during treatment is essential.

chloramphenicol A wide-range, orally active antibiotic but it is too toxic for general use. It is now used mainly in life-threatening infections where other drugs are unsuitable, and in typhoid fever. *Dose:* 2g daily, but in severe infections, 50mg/kg daily by intravenous injection. In pyogenic meningitis in children, 50–100mg/kg by injection daily may be required. Care is necessary when giving chloramphenicol to infants as it may cause the so-called 'grey syndrome'. Side-effects include nausea, neuritis and aplastic anaemia. Chloromycetin is also used locally in skin, eye and ear infections.

chlordiazepoxide A benzodiazepine used mainly in the short-term treatment of anxiety, and in alcoholism. *Dose:* 30mg daily, increased in severe anxiety up to 100mg daily, with half doses for elderly patients. Withdrawal of treatment should be gradual to avoid rebound effects. Side-effects include dizziness, drowsiness and ataxia. Prolonged use carries the risk of dependence.

chlorhexidine An antiseptic of high potency and a wide range of activity, although it is ineffective against spores and viruses. It is well tolerated by the tissues. For pre-operative skin preparation, a 0.5% solution in alcohol is often used; an aqueous solution (0.05%) is employed for general topical application, and a mixture of chlorhexidine and cetrimide (Savlon) is used when a detergent action is also required. Chlorhexidine is also used as a 1/10 000 (0.01%) solution for bladder irrigation, as it is effective against most urinary pathogens. A general-purpose cream and an obstetric cream are also available. Solutions of chlorhexidine and other antiseptics may become contaminated with *Pseudomonas*, and all aqueous solutions should be sterilized.

chlormethiazole A sedative with anticonvulsant properties. *Dose:* in severe insomnia in the elderly, 200–400mg orally; in alcohol withdrawal conditions, 400–

800mg initially, reduced and withdrawn over a 9-day period. It may also be given by intravenous infusion as a 0.8% solution. Chlormethiazole has also been given by injection in status epilepticus and the toxaemia of pregnancy in doses according to need and response. Side-effects are sneezing, gastro-intestinal disturbances and headache.

chlormezanone A minor tranquillizer similar to meprobamate, with some muscle-relaxant action. It is useful in anxiety states as well as in conditions associated with muscle spasm. *Dose:* 600–800mg daily with half doses for elderly patients. It has the sedative and other side-effects of anxiolytic drugs.

chloroform Once widely used as a general anaesthetic, but now obsolete. Used as chloroform-water in mixtures as a preservative and flavouring agent, and for its carminative effects.

chloroquine An antimalarial drug effective against the erythrocytic forms of most types of malarial parasites, and used for both prophylaxis and treatment of benign and malignant tertian malaria. It should be noted that chloroquine-resistant strains of *Plasmodium falciparum* are becoming increasingly common in SE Asia, Central and South America, and some other areas, and a return to treatment with quinine may be necessary. *Dose:* adult prophylaxis, 300mg once a week; for treatment of an attack of malaria, 600mg initially, followed by 300mg daily for 2–3 days. Seriously ill or vomiting patients should be given 200–300mg by intramuscular or slow intravenous injection, repeated once if necessary before oral treatment can be tolerated. Other dosage schemes are also in use, and for details reference should be made to standard works on the treatment of malaria. As chloroquine is concentrated in the liver, it has also been used in hepatic amoebiasis, but metronidazole is now often preferred. Chloroquine also has an action in rheumatoid inflammatory conditions similar to that of penicillamine, *Dose:* 150mg daily after food. Such use requires care, as extended therapy is necessary, and the drug may cause corneal opacity and irreversible retinal damage. Other side-effects are gastro-intestinal disturbances, rash and pruritus.

chlorothiazide The first of the thiazide diuretics, now largely replaced by bendrofluazide and similar drugs. *Dose:* 1–2g daily in oedematous states;

0.5–1g daily in hypertension. Potassium supplements may be necessary with extended treatment. See page 199.

chloroxylenol A germicide used in many non-caustic antiseptics. Although effective against streptococci, it is less active against staphylococci, and of no value against *Ps. aeruginosa* or *Proteus*.

chlorpheniramine A potent antihistamine with the action, uses and side-effects of the group, including drowsiness. *Dose:* 16–24mg daily: 10–20mg by intramuscular or subcutaneous injection as required. Doses of 10mg are sometimes added to intravenous drip solutions.

chlorpromazine A powerful tranquillizer or anti-psychotic agent with a wide range of activity on the central nervous system. It is widely used in the treatment of schizophrenia and other psychoses, in agitation and tension, and the management of refractory patients. It is also effective as an anti-emetic in terminal illness; in the short-term treatment of severe anxiety, and for the control of intractable hiccup. *Dose:* initially 75mg orally daily, slowly increased as required. In psychotic states, up to 1g daily. Single doses of 25–50mg may be given by *deep* i.m. injection in acute conditions. Suppositories of 100mg are also available. Side-effects include extrapyramidal and anticholinergic symptoms, drowsiness, hypotension, weight gain, rash, jaundice and haemolytic anaemia. Prolonged use may cause pigmentation of the skin and eyes. Care is necessary in hepatic and renal dysfunction. Skin sensitization may occur after contact with solutions of chlorpromazine.

chlorpropamide A long-acting hypoglycaemic agent of the sulphonylurea type. It is effective only if some insulin-secreting cells are still functional. It is used mainly in the treatment of mild diabetes mellitus occurring in middle-aged patients not responding to dietary control. Its long action makes it unsuitable for elderly diabetics. *Dose:* 250–500mg daily as a single morning dose. Side-effects are rash, jaundice, blood dyscrasia and hypoglycaemia, but are uncommon with low doses. Flushing may occur if alcohol is taken. Chlorpropamide (but not other sulphonylureas) is sometimes used to check the polyuria of diabetes insipidus. It acts by sensitizing the renal tubules to endogenous vasopressin, but great care is necessary to avoid hypoglycaemic reactions. *Dose:* up to 350mg daily in adults, or 200mg daily in children. See page 187.

chlortetracycline An orally effective antibiotic with the actions, uses and side-effects of the tetracyclines. *Dose:* 1–2g daily.

chlorthalidone A diuretic similar in action and uses to bendrofluazide, but with a longer duration of activity that permits a single morning dose. It is also useful in diabetes insipidus. *Dose:* as diuretic 50–100mg daily or on alternate days; in hypertension 25–50mg; up to 350mg daily in diabetes insipidus.

cholecalciferol See Vitamin D.

cholestyramine An exchange resin that binds with bile acids in the intestines and prevents their absorption. Such acids are essential for cholesterol synthesis, and resin-binding leading indirectly to a lowering of plasma cholesterol levels. *Dose:* in hyperlipidaemia: 12–24g daily, with water. It is also used in doses of 4–8g daily to relieve the pruritus associated with biliary obstruction. Side-effects are rash and gastro-intestinal disturbances. Cholestyramine and related agents may interfere with the absorption of anticoagulants and other drugs. See page 197.

choline theophyllinate A bronchodilator with the actions, uses and side-effects of aminophylline. *Dose:* 400–1600mg daily, after food.

chorionic gonadotrophin A gonad-stimulating hormone prepared from the urine of pregnancy. It has been used in anovulatory sterility, metropathia haemorrhagica, habitual abortion, and undescended testis. *Dose:* 500–1000 units by i.m. injection. Nausea, vomiting and oedema are side-effects.

chymotrypsin A proteolytic enzyme of the pancreas used in ophthalmology to facilitate intracapsular lens extraction.

cilastatin See imipenem.

cilazapril A long-acting ACE inhibitor with the actions, uses and side-effects of that group of drugs. *Dose:* in essential hypertension 1mg daily initially, increased up to 5mg daily according to need. In renovascular hypertension 0.25–0.5mg daily.

cimetidine A widely used selective histamine H_2 receptor antagonist. Unlike ordinary antihistamines, it inhibits gastric secretion, and is used in the treatment of peptic ulcer and other conditions of gastric hyperacidity. *Dose:* 800mg daily for at least 4 weeks. Dose by intramuscular or slow intravenous injection 200mg, 4–6 hourly. In stress ulceration, as much as 2.4g daily have been given. The dose should be reduced in renal impairment. The drug may increase the effects of oral anticoagulants and phenytoin. Side-effects include diarrhoea, rash and dizziness. It has some anti-androgen activity, and gynaecomastia is an occasional side-effect.

cinnarizine An antihistamine, chiefly of value in Ménière's disease, although it is also used in travel sickness and in peripheral vascular disorders. *Dose:* 45–90mg daily. Drowsiness and gastrointestinal disturbances are side-effects.

cinoxacin A quinolone derivative with actions, uses and side-effects similar to those of nalidixic acid. *Dose:* in urinary tract infections, 1g daily; prophylaxis 500mg daily. Contra-indicated in severe renal impairment.

ciprofloxacin A quinolone with a wide range of activity against both Gram-positive and Gram-negative bacteria, including *Pseudomonas* and *Proteus*. It is effective in many systemic infections, as well as in bone, joint and urinary infections, and in gonorrhoea, but is indicated mainly in infections resistant to other antibacterial agents. *Dose:* 500mg–1.5g daily for 5–7 days; in gonorrhoea, a single dose of 250mg is given. In severe infections 200–400mg daily by intravenous infusion for 5–7 days. Side-effects include nausea, dizziness, headache, rash and pruritus. Plasma levels of theophylline may be increased and should be closely controlled. Care is necessary in convulsive disorders.

cisapride A gastro-intestinal stimulant with an action that appears to be mediated by the release of acetylcholine, as its effects can be inhibited by drugs such as atropine. It is given to relieve gastro-oesophageal reflux and delayed gastric emptying. *Dose:* 30–40mg daily before meals, and at night, for some weeks. Side-effects are abdominal pain and diarrhoea. Unlike metoclopramide, it has no central anti-emetic properties.

cisplatin A cytotoxic agent containing platinum bound in an organic complex. The action is linked with drug-induced changes in DNA structure that inhibit cell development. It is used in ovarian, testicular and other solid tumours, and in resistant malignant conditions, sometimes in association with other antineoplastic agents. *Dose:* by intravenous injection, 15–20mg/m^2 daily for 5 days a month, or 50–120mg/m^2 monthly. Blood tests are essential throughout treatment. Side-effects, which may be severe, include nausea, vomiting, and oto-, nephro-, and myelotoxicity.

clarithromycin A macrolide antibiotic similar to erythromycin, but with better absorption and reduced gastro-intestinal side-effects. *Dose:* 250mg twice a day for 7 days, doubled in severe infections. Care in heptic and renal impairment. It may potentiate the effects of warfarin and digoxin.

clavulanic acid An inhibitor of beta-lactamase. Many penicillin-resistant organisms contain that enzyme in the cell wall, which inactivates the penicillin before it can enter the cell and exert its bacterial action. Clavulanic acid inhibits such enzyme activity, and so facilitates the penetration of the antibiotic into the bacterial cell. It is used in association with amoxycillin as co-amoxiclav (Augmentin) and with ticarcillin, as Timentin, in the treatment of infections due to amoxycillin-resistant bacteria.

clemastine An antihistamine used in allergic rhinitis, urticaria and allergic dermatoses. *Dose:* 1mg twice a day. In common with other antihistamines, it may cause drowsiness, and anticholinergic side-effects such as dryness of the mouth.

clindamycin An antibiotic with a range of activity similar to erythromycin, but it is used mainly in staphylococcal bone and joint infections not responding to other drugs. It is also useful in anaerobic abdominal infections. *Dose:* 600–1800mg daily. It is also used as an alternative to erythromycin in doses of 600mg before dentistry in infective endocarditis. A serious side-effect is a potentially fatal pseudomembranous colitis, and the drug should be withdrawn immediately if diarrhoea occurs. See vancomycin and metronidazole. It is used locally as a 1% solution in acne.

clobazam A benzodiazepine tranquillizer with the actions and uses of diazepam, but with reduced sedative effects. It is used mainly in the short-term treatment of anxiety. *Doses:* 20–30mg as a single nightly dose. In severe anxiety larger but divided doses may be given under medical control. It is also useful in the auxiliary treatment of epilepsy.

clobetasol A potent corticosteroid used as cream or ointment (0.05%) in the short-term treatment of severe inflammatory skin conditions not responding to less powerful drugs. The application should be used sparingly as absorption with systematic and local side-effects may occur with excessive or prolonged treatment.

clobetasone A locally acting corticosteroid, used as cream or ointment (0.05%) in eczema and inflammatory skin conditions not responding to less potent corticosteroids.

clofazimine An antileprotic agent given in association with dapsone to prevent the incidence of resistance. *Dose:* 300mg monthly; in lepra reactions, 300mg daily for three months. It may cause discoloration of the urine, skin and lesions.

clofibrate A plasma-lipid regulating agent used in hyperlipid aemia, in conjunction with dietary measures, to reduce excessive plasma levels of cholesterol and triglycerides. *Dose:* 2g daily, with regular checks on plasma lipid levels. Side-effects are transient nausea and abdominal discomfort. It increases the biliary excretion of cholesterol, and gall stones are a contra-in dication. A myositis-like reaction may occur in renal impairment, and the drug should be withdrawn. See also page 197. Clofibrate may potentiate the action of oral anticoagulants, the dose of which may require adjustment.

clomiphene An anti-oestrogen used to stimulate ovulation in some types of anovulatory sterility. *Dose:* 50mg daily for 5 days a month, repeated if ovulation does not occur. Its use has resulted in occasional multiple births. If pregnancy does not follow up to six courses, further treatment is of little use. Side-effects are hot flushes and abdominal discomfort; visual disturbances indicate that treatment should be withdrawn. Contra-indicated in hepatic disease and ovarian neoplasm.

clomipramine A tricyclic antidepressant with the actions, uses and side-effects of imipramine and related drugs, but with reduced sedative properties. *Dose:* 30–150mg daily orally; up to 150mg daily by intramuscular injection.

clomocycline A derivative of tetracyline, with similar actions and uses. *Dose:* 510–1360mg daily (3–8 capsules).

clonazepam A benzodiazepine, with a marked anticonvulsant action of value in all types of epilepsy. *Dose:* 1mg daily initially, increased up to 8mg daily according to need. In status epilepticus, 1mg by slow intravenous injection, but apnoea and hypotension, requiring prompt treatment, may occur. Side-effects include drowsiness, dizziness and irritability and, occasionally, paradoxical aggression.

clonidine A centrally-acting antihypertensive agent, now used less frequently. *Dose:* 150–300μg daily initially, increased if required up to 1.2mg daily. Doses up to 300μg have been given by slow intravenous injection. Sudden withdrawal of the drug may provoke a hypertensive crisis. Clonidine is also used in doses of 100μg daily in the prophylaxis of migraine, and to alleviate menopausal flushing. The side-effects include sedation, dry mouth, fluid retention and bradycardia.

clopenthixol See zuclopenthixol.

clorazepate A benzodiazepine tranquillizer with the actions, uses and side-effects of diazepam. Used mainly in the short-term treatment of anxiety. *Dose:* 7.5–22.5mg daily, or a single dose of 15mg at night.

clotrimazole An antifungal agent used locally in vaginal candidiasis. *Dose:* 100–200mg as vaginal tablets or pessaries for nightly insertion. Also used as a 1% cream, lotion or dusting powder for fungal infections of the skin and ears. Side-effects are local irritation and erythema.

cloxacillin An acid-stable, semi-synthetic penicillin that is not broken down by the enzyme penicillinase, and so is effective in infections due to penicillin-resistant staphylococci. *Dose:* 2g daily before food. In severe infections, 250–500mg by injection 6-hourly. Now largely replaced by flucloxacillin. The side-effects are those of the penicillins generally.

clozapine A new potent but potentially toxic dopamine-receptor blocking agent used in schizophrenia resistant to other drugs. *Dose:* 25–50mg daily initially, slowly increased to 300mg daily according to need. A serious side-effect is neutropenia that may lead to agranulocytosis, and treatment must be under hospital supervision with regular blood monitoring. Patient, doctor and hospital pharmacist must be registered with the Clozaril (clozapine) Patient Monitoring Service to maintain the necessary strict control of treatment.

coal tar The black viscous liquid obtained from the distillation of coal. It is used mainly as Zinc and Tar Paste in eczema, psoriasis and pruritus.

co-amilofruse A mixture of the diuretics amiloride and frusemide.

co-amilozide A mixture of the diuretics amiloride and hydrochlorothiazide.

co-amoxiclav A mixture of clavulanic acid and amoxycillin. The resistance to penicillin by staphylococci and other organisms is due to penicillinases such as beta-lactamase in the bacterial cell wall. Those enzymes inactivate penicillin before it can enter the cell and exert its antibacterial action. Such inactivation can be prevented by inhibitors of beta-lactamase such as clavulanic acid. That acid has no anti-bacterial action, but when given with a penicillin the antibiotic is able to penetrate into the cell without loss of activity. The combination is of value in infections due to penicillin-resistant-penicillinase-producing bacteria, including most staphylococci. *Dose:* as amoxycillin 750mg daily, doubled in severe infections, or 3–4g daily by slow intravenous injection.

co-beneldopa A mixture of levodopa and benzerazide. See levodopa.

†**cocaine** A local anaesthetic. Still used occasionally in ophthalmology as a 2% solution, often with homatropine, *q.v.*

co-careldopa A mixture of levodopa and carbidopa. See levodopa.

co-codamol Codeine, with paracetamol.

co-codaprin Codeine, with aspirin.

co-danthramer Danthron, with poloxamer.

cod-liver oil A rich source of vitamins A and D. It is used as a dietary supplement to improve general nutrition, promote calcification and prevent rickets. *Dose:* 2–10ml daily.

codeine One of the alkaloids of opium. It depresses the cough centre and is used in the treatment of useless cough. It also reduces intestinal motility, and is useful in the symptomatic treatment of diarrhoea. It also has mild analgesic properties, and is present with aspirin in co-codaprin, Veganin, and similar preparations. In large doses the constipating action of codeine may be a disadvantage. *Dose:* 10–60mg.

co-dergocrine A cerebral vasodilator, sometimes used in the treatment of senile dementia. *Dose:* 4.5mg daily, but the response is unreliable. Side-effects include nausea, rash and bradycardia.

co-dydramol Dihydrocodeine, with paracetamol.

co-fluampicil A mixture of flucloxacillin and ampicillin.

co-flumactone A mixture of spironolactone and hydrochlorothiazide.

colchicine The alkaloid obtained from meadow saffron. It is used in acute gout. *Dose:* 500μg every 2 hours until relief is obtained. A total dose of 10mg should not be exceeded, but relief of pain or the onset of vomiting or diarrhoea usually renders full doses unnecessary. It is also used prophylactically in doses of 500μg two or three times a day during early treatment with allopurinol, probenecid and sulphinpyrazone. Care is necessary in the elderly, and in renal impairment.

colestipol An exchange resin used in hyperlipidaemia that acts by binding with bile salts in the gut, prevents their reabsorption, and so indirectly lowers the plasma level of cholesterol. See page 197. *Dose:* 10–30g daily. May interfere with the absorption of many drugs.

colfosceril A surface-tension lowering agent for relieving the respiratory syndrome in premature babies. It is given via the endotracheal tube in mechanically ventilated infants under expert control.

colistin An antibiotic chiefly effective against Gram-negative organisms and used mainly for bowel sterilization. *Dose:* 4.5–9 mega units daily. In systemic infections 2 mega units 8-hourly by injection have been used, but less toxic antibiotics are now preferred.

collodion Pyroxylin, dissolved in a mixture of alcohol and ether. When applied to the skin, it dries to form a flexible film, and it is used to seal minor cuts and abrasions. It is also used as a vehicle for the extended local application of drugs such as salicylic acid, *q.v.*

congo red A red dye formerly used by intravenous injection as a 1% solution in the diagnosis of amyloid disease.

Coparvax A preparation of inactivated *Corynebacterium parvum* organisms. It is used by injection into the pleural or peritoneal cavity (after aspiration) in the treatment of malignant pleural effusion and malignant ascites. *Dose:* 7–14mg, repeated if necessary after 7 days. Nausea, fever and abdominal pain are side-effects.

co-phenotrope A mixture of diphenoxylate and atropine.

co-prenozide A mixture of oxprenolol and cyclopenthiazide.

co-proxamol A mixture of dextropropoxyphene and paracetamol.

copper sulphate The main constituent of Clinitest tablets and Benedict's solution used for testing for glucose in urine.

corticosteroids Hormones secreted by the cortex of the suprarenal gland. The principal hormone is hydrocortisone but more potent synthetic derivatives such as dexamethasone are also available.

corticotrophin The adrenocorticotrophic hormone of the anterior pituitary gland. It stimulates the production of corticosteroid hormones by the adrenal cortex. It has been used as an alternative to the corticosteroids, but it is now used mainly as a test of adrenocortical function, as following intramuscular injection, the plasma level of hydrocortisone normally rises. See tetracosactrin.

cortisol Hydrocortisone.

cortisone One of the corticosteroids secreted by the adrenal cortex. Although it is rapidly absorbed orally, it is inactive until converted in the liver to hydrocortisone. It therefore has the actions, uses and side-effects of hydrocortisone, which is often the preferred corticosteroid. It should be noted that cortisone is of no value for topical application. See hydrocortisone and table of corticosteroids, page 267.

co-tenidone A mixture of atenolol and chlorthalidone.

co-trimoxazole A mixture of trimethoprim and sulphamethoxazole. Trimethaprim, like the sulphonamides, interferes with the folic acid cycle of bacterial metabolism, but at a different point, and the mixture has an increased antibacterial action. It is used in urinary tract infections, bronchitis, salmonella infections, and typhoid fever, and in high doses against *Pneumocystitis carinii* infections. *Dose:* 960mg 12-hrly, orally or by injection, doubled in severe infections. In *Pneumocystitis carinii* infections 120mg/kg daily for 14 days. The side-effects of co-trimoxazole are those of its constituents. There is a trend towards giving trimethaprim alone in some infections, as co-trimoxazole may be too toxic for elderly patients.

coumarins Compounds that depress the formation in the liver of prothrombin and other blood coagulation factors. They are used in the prevention and treatment of venous thrombosis and pulmonary embolism, and to prevent the development of clots on heart valve implants. Unlike heparin, they are active orally. The dose is based on the degree of prothrombin activity in the blood and, as the onset of treatment is slow, initial therapy often includes the concurrent use of a few doses of heparin. The coumarins should be used with care in hypertension, and in renal and hepatic insufficiency. The main risk of overdose is haemorrhage, and an early sign is bleeding from the gums. They are not indicated in arterial or cerebral thrombosis. See warfarin and phenindione.

counter-irritants Substances, also referred to as rubifacients that, when applied to the skin, produce a mild, local irritation and inflammation. Such a rubifacient action, which follows stimulation of the nerves of the unbroken skin, gives symptomatic relief in painful conditions of the muscles and joints. Creams and liniments containing methyl salicylate, turpentine, capsicum resin and menthol are examples of rubifacients.

crisantaspase Asparagine is an aminoacid essential for the development of some malignant cells. Crisantaspase is an enzyme, also known as asparaginase, that breaks down asparagine, and so has an indirect cytotoxic action. It is used to induce remission in acute lymphoblastic leukaemia in children. *Dose* (after pre-treatment with other drugs): 1000 units/kg by slow intravenous injection daily for ten days. Side-effects include anaphylactic reactions, and skin tests to detect hypersensitivity are essential before initial and re-treatment.

crotamiton An ascaricide and antipruritic. Used by local application as cream or lotion (10%) in the treatment of scabies and itching conditions.

crystal violet A dyestuff with a selective action against Gram-positive organisms and yeasts. Formerly used as a 0.5% solution for infected skin conditions, and an alcoholic solution with brilliant green is used for skin preparation.

cyanocobalamin The anti-anaemic factor present in liver. It is specific in the treatment of pernicious anaemia and its neurological complications, and of value in some other anaemias due to nutritional deficiencies. *Dose:* in pernicious anaemia, 1mg by intramuscular injection at monthly intervals. It has been largely replaced by hydroxocobalamin, which has a more prolonged action.

cyclandelate A vasodilator used in peripheral circulatory disorders such as acrocyanosis and vasospasm, and in cerebrovascular disease. *Dose:* 1.2–1.6g daily. Side-effects include nausea, flushing and dizziness.

cyclizine An antihistamine, used mainly in travel sickness and nausea generally. Also useful in vertigo. *Dose:* 100–150mg daily. Side-effects include dryness of the mouth, headache and drowsiness.

cyclofenil An anti-oestrogen with the actions and uses of clomiphene. *Dose:* 200mg twice a day for 10 days for three menstrual cycles. Hot flushes and abdominal discomfort are side-effects.

cyclopenthiazide A thiazide diuretic with the actions, uses and side-effects of bendrofluazide. *Dose:* 1mg initially, 250–500μg daily or on alternate days, in the morning, according to need.

cyclopentolate An anticholinergic agent used to produce cycloplegia and mydriasis. The action is more rapid and less prolonged than atropine, particularly in children.

cyclophosphamide A widely used alkylating cytotoxic

agent, active orally and by injection. Used in Hodgkin's disease, chronic lymphocytic leukaemia and lymphomas. *Dose:* 100–300mg daily, orally or intravenously, or 500mg–1g weekly. A high fluid intake is necessary, as a metabolite may cause haemorrhagic cystitis, and it is sometimes used with mesna to reduce the risk of such cystitis. Nausea and vomiting are common side-effects, as is epilation with high doses.

cyclopropane An inhalation anaesthetic of high potency with which induction and recovery are rapid. It causes some respiratory depression and cardiac irregularities, and its administration requires care. It is used with closed-circuit apparatus as it forms an explosive mixture with air and oxygen. Supplied in orange-coloured cylinders.

cycloserine An antibiotic used in pulmonary tuberculosis when standard drugs are ineffective. Occasionally used in urinary infections. *Dose:* 250–750mg daily. Side-effects include drowsiness, vertigo and rash.

cyclosporin An antibiotic with a powerful immunosuppressant action. It is used under expert control to prevent graft rejection in organ and bone marrow transplantation, and in the prevention of graft-versus-host disease (GVHD). Prolonged therapy over some months may be required. Side-effects include tremor, gastrointestinal disturbance, hypertrichosis and nephrotoxicity.

cyproheptadine A compound with antihistamine and anti-serotonin properties. Some allergic reactions are due not only to histamine, but also to serotonin, and cyproheptadine is useful in conditions not responding completely to an antihistamine. *Dose:* 4–20mg daily. It has been used as an appetite stimulant in doses of 12mg daily.

cyproterone An anti-androgen used to reduce libido in sexual deviants. *Dose:* 50–100mg daily. It is also used in the palliative treatment of prostatic carcinoma, particularly in advanced cases that have become resistant to other therapy. *Dose:* 300mg daily. For severe, refractory acne in females, 2mg daily with ethinyloestradiol. Side-effects are fatigue and lassitude, weight gain and gynaecomastia. Contra-indicated in severe depression and acute hepatic disease. Care is necessary in diabetics.

cytarabine A cytotoxic agent that prevents cell development by inhibiting the formation of nucleic acid. It is used mainly in the control of acute myeloblastic leukaemia. *Dose:* 0.5–3mg/kg daily by intravenous or subcutaneous injection. Close haematological control is essential as the drug is a powerful myelodepressant. Other side-effects are those of the cytotoxic drugs, generally, but fever, myalgia and bone pain may also occur.

cytotoxic drugs A term applied to drugs that can kill cancer cells. In practice, many factors influence their therapeutic value. They are rarely selective, and therapeutic doses usually have a toxic effect on some normal cells. They may attack cancer cells at different stages of development, as actively dividing cells are more susceptible than resting cells. They may not reach the cancer cells in adequate concentration, or resistance to the drug may develop. The dose may also depend to some extent on the patient's tolerance of the drug, and combined treatment with two or more drugs may have the advantages of increased potency with reduced toxicity. All cytotoxic drugs, with the exception of bleomycin and vincristine, bring about a depression of the bone marrow, which may be severe, and some degree of hair loss, which is usually reversible. Severe nausea and vomiting are also common, and early use of powerful anti-emetics is essential. Many cytotoxic agents are tissue irritants, and with intravenous treatment great care must be taken to avoid extravasation, as severe local tissue damage can occur. See alkylating agents and antimetabolites. See pages 180–182.

D

dacarbazine A cytotoxic drug that appears to depress purine metabolism and the formation of DNA. It is used mainly in malignant melanoma, and in combination with other agents it is of value in other malignant conditions. *Dose:* 2.5–4.5mg/kg, daily for 10 days, repeated after 4 weeks. Side-effects are severe nausea, bone marrow depression and an influenza-like syndrome. The drug should be handled with care, as it is a tissue irritant.

dactinomycin See Actinomycin D.

danazol A derivative of ethisterone that inhibits the release of pituitary gonadotrophins. Used in conditions such as endometriosis, gynaecomastia and precocious puberty. *Dose:* 100–400mg daily, starting during menstruation. Side-effects are nausea, dizziness, rash, flushing and hair loss. Care is necessary in cardiac, renal or hepatic impairment, and in epilepsy and diabetes.

danthron A synthetic anthraquinone laxative used mainly for constipation in the aged, and in drug-induced constipation in the terminally ill. Not suitable for routine use by other patients. It is given in doses of 25–25mg as co-danthamer, and acts within 6–12 hrs. The urine may be coloured red.

dantrolene A skeletal muscle relaxant that acts on the muscle fibre, and not at the myoneural junction. The action may be linked with an interference with the movement of calcium ions. It is used in the severe and chronic spastic states that occur after stroke, spinal cord injury, and in multiple sclerosis. *Dose:* 25mg daily initially, increased at weekly intervals up to a maximum of 400mg daily after 7 weeks, as the response is slow and may be inadequate. The side-effects of weakness and fatigue are mild, and often transient, but liver function tests during treatment are essential. Dantrolene is also of value in malignant hyperthermia, a rare but serious complication of anaesthesia, and is given in doses of 1mg/kg by intravenous injection as soon as the condition is diagnosed, and repeated up to a total of 10mg/kg.

dapsone A sulphone compound used in the treatment of leprosy. *Dose:* 25–400mg orally twice weekly in leprosy, and continued for some years. Resistance to dapsone may occur, and combined treatment with clofazimine and rifampicin may be necessary. Dapsone is sometimes given with pyrimethamine in chloroquine-resistant malaria. Side-effects are nausea, rash, neuropathy and myelodepression.

debrisoquine An adrenergic neurone blocking agent with the actions, uses and side-effects of guanethidine, except that it is less likely to cause diarrhoea. It is used mainly in resistant hypertension, in association with other drugs.

dehydrocholic acid A stimulant of biliary secretion used orally to disperse small calculi in the bile duct, and to increase the elimination of contrast agents from the gall bladder. *Dose:* 750–2250mg daily; in cholecystography, 500–750mg 4-hrly for 12 hours before and after X-ray visualization. Contra-indicated in chronic liver disease.

demeclocycline An antibiotic with the actions, uses and side-effects of tetracycline, but more likely to cause photo-allergic reactions. *Dose:* 600mg daily.

dequalinium A mild anti-infective agent used as pastilles or lozenges containing 250μg for oro-pharyngeal infections.

desferrioxamine A chelating agent that combines with iron salts to form a soluble non-toxic complex. Of great value in acute ferrous sulphate poisoning in children. *Dose:* 2g immediately by intramuscular injection, together with gastric lavage (2g of desferrioxamine/l) followed by a single oral dose of 10g. It may also be given by continuous intravenous infusion, 15mg/kg hrly up to a maximum of 80mg/kg. It may cause hypotension if the infusion is given too rapidly. It is also useful in the treatment of iron-overload caused by repeated blood transfusions, and for aluminium overload in patients on dialysis.

desipramine A derivative of imipramine, with similar anti-depressant properties, but with a more rapid action. A response may be apparent within a week of treatment. *Dose:* 25–75mg, sometimes as a single dose at night, increasing to 200mg daily as required.

desmopressin A derivative of vasopressin, with increased potency and longer duration of action. Used in the diagnosis and control of diabetes insipidus, and in the treatment of nocturnal enuresis. *Dose:* 10–20μg intranasally once or twice a day; 1–4μg daily by injection.

desonide A powerful locally acting corticosteroid, used in eczema and other severe skin conditions not responding to less potent corticosteroids. Cream and ointment contain 0.05%.

desoxymethasone A corticosteroid, for local application in acute inflammatory and allergic skin conditions. Used as oily cream 0.25%.

dexamethasone A potent synthetic corticosteroid, with reduced salt-retaining properties. Useful in all conditions requiring systemic corticosteroid therapy (except Addison's disease), including inflammatory and allergic disorders, shock, cerebral oedema, and adrenal hyperplasia. *Dose:* 0.5–2mg daily up to a maximum of 15mg daily; in shock, 2–6mg/kg by slow intravenous injection or infusion; in cerebral oedema, 10mg initially by intravenous injection, followed by 4mg i.m. 6-hrly. Dexamethasone is also given by intra-articular injection for local inflammation of joints in doses of 0.4–4mg. It is also used as eye-drops (0.01%) in uveitis, but care is necessary, with prolonged treatment as with some patients a 'steroid glaucoma' may be precipitated.

†**dexamphetamine sulphate** A central nervous system stimulant. It is used in the treatment of narcolepsy and, paradoxically, it is sometimes useful in hyperkinesia in children. *Dose:* in narcolepsy, 20–60mg daily; in hyperkinesia 2.5mg initially, slowly increased up to a maximum of 20mg daily. Side-effects are insomnia, anorexia and agitation. Dependence and tolerance may occur early.

dexfenfluramine An appetite depressant closely related to fenfluramine. *Dose:* 30mg daily. Weight reduction develops after 2 weeks, but treatment should not extend beyond 3 months. It may potentiate the action of antihypertensive agents, antidiabetics and sedatives. Side-effects are dry mouth and gastro-intestinal disturbances.

dextran A blood-plasma substitute obtained from sucrose solutions by bacterial action, and used as solutions of varying molecular weight (dextran 40, 70, 110). Dextrans 70 and 110 are used as blood volume expanders by intravenous injection in some cases of shock, and dextran 40 is used mainly to improve post-operative peripheral circulation and reduce blood viscosity, and to prevent thrombo-embolism. Care must be taken to adjust dose to avoid overloading the circulation. Any blood-matching should be carried out before giving dextran.

dextromethorphan A cough centre depressant with the actions and uses of pholcodine.

†**dextromoramide** A powerful synthetic analgesic with a shorter and less sedating action than morphine. Of value in severe and intractable pain, and in terminal disease. *Dose:* 5mg, or more, either orally or by injection, according to need and response. Care is necessary in liver dysfunction and respiratory depression.

dextropropoxyphene An orally effective analgesic present in co-proxamol. Of value in many painful conditions, and in malignant disease its use may delay the need to resort to the opiate analgesics. *Dose:* 250mg, or more, daily, but doses in excess of 700mg daily may cause toxic psychoses and convulsions.

dextrose Glucose.

†**diamorphine** A derivative of morphine with a more powerful analgesic and cough-suppressant action. It is also less liable to cause nausea. Valuable for the relief of severe pain and the suppression of useless cough. Addiction is a constant risk owing to the euphoric effects of the drug. *Dose:* 5–10mg orally or

by injection, repeated as required. For severe pain in the terminally ill, addiction is of no consequence, and much larger doses are given according to need: if necessary, by continuous infusion or a syringe-pump device.

diazepam A benzodiazepine, of value in anxiety states, insomnia, acute alcoholic withdrawal, and for premedication. It has a muscle relaxant action, and is valuable when given by injection in status epilepticus and in the control of the spasm of tetanus. *Doses:* 5–30mg daily, 2–10mg by slow intravenous injection as required, up to a maximum of 30mg in 8 hrs. Absorption after intramuscular injection is slow and unreliable. It is sometimes given as suppositories of 5–10mg. Side-effects are drowsiness, dizziness, respiratory depression and hypersensitivity reactions. Care is necessary in glaucoma and renal and hepatic impairment. Extended treatment may lead to dependence and addiction, and withdrawal should be slow to avoid the risks of precipitating toxic psychosis, confusion and convulsions.

diazoxide An inhibitor of insulin secretion given orally in doses of 5mg/kg or more daily in severe hypoglycaemia. Also of value in severe hypertensive crisis, in doses up to 150mg by rapid intravenous injection. Side-effects are nausea, tachycardia and oedema.

dichlorphenamide An inhibitor of carbonic anhydrase, used in the treatment of glaucoma as it lowers the intra-ocular pressure by reducing the sodium bicarbonate content of the aqueous humour. It is sometimes used as a mild diuretic. *Dose:* 200mg daily. Side-effects are paraesthesia, drowsiness and depression.

diclofenac A non-steroidal anti-inflammatory drug (NSAID) of the naproxen type, and used in rheumatoid, arthritic and similar conditions. *Dose:* 75–150mg daily, after food. Suppositories of 100mg are useful at night, but may cause local irritation. In acute conditions, and in ureteric colic, 75mg by deep intramuscular injection. Like other NSAIDs, diclofenac may cause gastric disturbance and hypersensitivity reactions. See page 214.

dicobalt edetate A specific antidote in acute cyanide poisoning; toxic in other conditions. *Dose:* 300mg by slow intravenous injection, followed by 50ml of glucose solution 50%, repeated if required.

dicyclomine An anticholinergic agent used to reduce gastric hyperacidity and the smooth muscle spasm of gastrointestinal disorders. *Dose:* 30–60mg daily. Side-effects include dryness of the mouth and blurred vision.

dienoestrol A synthetic oestrogen similar to stilboestrol, but used mainly as a 0.025% cream for senile or atrophic vaginitis.

diethylcarbamazine A synthetic drug used in filariasis but long-term treatment is necessary. *Dose:* 1mg/kg daily initially, slowly increased to 6mg/kg daily, and continued for 21 days. Low initial doses are necessary to reduce allergic reactions due to proteins released from dead worms. Side-effects include headache, nausea, rash and conjunctivitis. See ivermectin.

†**diethylpropion** An appetite-depressant related chemically to the amphetamines, but with reduced central stimulant effects. *Dose:* in the short-term treatment of obesity, 75mg daily for not longer than 8 weeks. Dependence may occur with prolonged treatment and the use of the drug is no longer recommended.

diflucortolone A corticosteroid, used topically as a 0.1% or 0.3% cream or ointment in steroid-responsive dermatoses. Of value in resistant conditions.

diflunisal An anti-inflammatory and analgesic drug (NSAID), chemically related to aspirin, but with actions and uses similar to naproxen. Dose: 500mg–1g daily. Care is necessary in aspirin-sensitive patients, and in peptic ulcer.

Digibind A highly purified preparation of sheep-derived digoxin-specific antibodies, given by intravenous infusion in digoxin and digitoxin overdose or poisoning. It mobilizes digoxin from cardiac receptor sites and binds it as an inert complex which is excreted in the urine, and symptoms of digoxin toxicity subside within an hour. The dose depends on the amount of digoxin absorbed; 40mg can neutralize about 600μg of digoxin.

digitalis The dried leaf of the foxglove, *Digitalis purpurea*. It has a powerful strengthening and regulatory action on the heart, but is now used as digoxin.

digitoxin The most powerful cardiac glycoside of digitalis leaf, of value in heart failure and atrial fibrillation. Absorption is rapid but excretion, which depends on metabolism by the liver, is very slow, and cumulative effects may occur. *Maintenance dose:* which requires careful adjustment, varies from 50–200μg daily.

digoxin The principal cardiac

glycoside obtained from digitalis leaf. It is rapidly absorbed orally, and is widely used in cardiac failure, paroxysmal tachycardia and atrial fibrillation. The diuresis of digoxin therapy is a secondary effect following on the improvement in the renal circulation. *Dose:* for rapid digitalization, 1–1.5mg initially over 24 hours; subsequent maintenance dose, 125–500μg daily. For slow digitalization, 250–500μg may be given daily for about a week, with subsequent doses based on the response. Elderly patients and children respond adequately to smaller doses, and tablets of 62.5μg (Lanoxin-PG) are available for such patients. In emergency, digoxin can be given by slow intravenous injection in doses of 0.75–1mg. Nausea and vomiting are often signs of overdose. If the heart rate falls below 60 beats per minute, dosage requires adjustment.

digoxin-specific antibody See Digibind.

dihydrocodeine An analgesic derived from codeine, but with a more powerful action. Of value in many painful conditions where mild analgesics are inadequate. *Dose:* 30mg orally after food, or 50mg by intramuscular or deep subcutaneous injection at intervals of 4–6 hrs according to need. Dizziness and constipation are side-effects.

dihydroergotamine A less potent derivative of ergotamine, with a similar antimigraine action and side-effects. *Dose:* 1mg by intramuscular or subcutaneous injection, repeated after 30 minutes as required. Maximum dose 3mg daily or 6mg a week. See page 194.

dihydrotachysterol A sterol related to calciferol, but with more rapid calcium-mobilizing properties. It is used mainly in hypocalcaemia and parathyroid tetany, but is sometimes effective in calciferol-resistant rickets. *Dose:* 200μg daily, adjusted to need according to plasma calcium levels.

diloxanide A well-tolerated amoebicide used in chronic intestinal amoebiasis when only cysts are present in the faeces. It is also used in acute infections, 5 days after a course of metronidazole. *Dose:* 1.5g daily for 10 days.

diltiazem A calcium-channel blocking agent, used in the prophylaxis and treatment of angina, and useful when beta-blocking agents are unsuitable or ineffective. *Dose:* 180–360mg daily, reduced in renal impairment. It may cause bradycardia, ankle oedema and rash.

dimenhydrinate An antihistamine used mainly as an

anti-emetic in nausea, trvel sickness and vertigo. *Dose:* 100–300mg daily. It may cause more drowsiness than some related drugs.

dimercaprol (BAL) A specific drug for the treatment of poisoning by arsenic, mercury, gold and other heavy metals. *Dose:* up to 3mg/kg 4-hrly by intramuscular injection for 2 days, gradually reduced to twice or once daily for 10 days. Side-effects include malaise, sweating, tachycardia, lachrymation and muscle spasm.

dimethicone Activated dimethicone is an antifoaming agent, said to reduce flatulence and protect mucous membranes. It is a constituent of many antacid preparations. It is also present in some water-repellent skin creams.

dimethindene An antihistamine with sedative properties used for the symptomatic relief of many allergic conditions. *Dose:* 5mg daily.

dimethylsulphoxide (DMSO) An organic solvent; used as a solvent for idoxuridine. It has also been used for the symptomatic relief of interstitial cystitis (Hunner's ulcer) by the bladder instillation of 50ml of a 50% solution.

dinoprost Prostaglandin $F_{2\alpha}$. It has actions and uses similar to dinoprostone.

dinoprostone A synthetic form of prostaglandin E_2. It initiates contractions of the pregnant uterus. *Dose:* 500μg orally to induce labour, repeated if necessary at hourly intervals; as vaginal tablets or gel, 3mg. Side-effects are nausea, diarrhoea, shivering and dizziness.

dioctyl sodium sulphosuccinate A slow-acting faecal softener. *Dose:* 500mg daily. See docusate.

diodone injection A solution of a complex organic iodine compound, used as a contrast agent in X-ray examination of kidneys and ureters.

diphenhydramine One of the early antihistamines, with a more sedative action than some newer compounds. It survives as a constitutent of some cough preparations and nasal decongestant products.

diphenoxylate A derivative of pethidine that resembles codeine in reducing intestinal activity. It is used for the symptomatic relief of diarrhoea, and is usually given with a small dose of atropine to discourage excessive dosage and to reduce the risk of dependence. *Dose:* 10mg initially, then 5mg every 6 hrs as required.

diphenylpyraline An antihistamine with actions, uses and side-effects similar to those of promethazine, but with reduced sedative effects. *Dose:* 5–20mg daily.

†**dipipanone** A rapidly acting

morphine-like analgesic of value in the severe pain of terminal disease. *Dose:* 30–360mg daily, but it is usually given in association with cyclizine as †Diconal. The side-effects are similar to those of morphine.

dipivefrin A pro-drug that is converted into adrenaline after absorption. It is used in chronic open angle glaucoma as eye-drops (0.1%).

dipyridamole An inhibitor of thrombus formation by reducing the adhesiveness of blood platelets, especially in the arterial circulation. *Dose:* 300–600mg daily before food. Side-effects include nausea, diarrhoea and headache.

disodium cromoglycate See sodium cromoglycate.

disodium edetate See sodium edetate, *q.v.*

disodium etidronate A diphosphonate that inhibits excessive bone demineralization. Of value in Paget's disease of the bone. *Dose:* 5mg/kg as a single daily dose for up to 6 months. Care is necessary in renal impairment. It is also given by intravenous infusion in malignant hypercalcaemia. *Dose:* 7.5mg/kg daily for 7 days; with oral maintenance doses of 20mg/kg daily as a single dose. Calcium-containing foods should be avoided within 2 hrs before or after treatment. Side-effects include nausea, diarrhoea, transient loss of taste and increase in bone pain.

disodium pamidronate A diphosphonate similar to disodium etidronate, but used in the single dose treatment of tumour-induced hypercalcaemia. The dose is based on the plasma calcium level, and varies from 15–60mg, given by slow intravenous infusion. The plasma calcium level soon falls, with a maximum lowering after 4–5 days. The response may be less effective after subsequent injections. A side-effect is a mild transient rise in body temperature. Care is necessary in renal impairment.

disopyramide A quinidine-like drug used in the treatment of cardiac arrhythmias especially after myocardial infarction. *Dose:* 300–800mg daily; dose by slow intravenous injection under ECG cover, 2mg/kg up to 150mg, followed by oral therapy as soon as possible. Care is necessary if a degree of heart block is present, and by its anticholinergic action, glaucoma and prostatic enlargement are contra-indications.

distigmine An inhibitor of cholinesterase similar to neostigmine but with a longer action. Dose in the control of myasthenia gravis 5–20mg as a single morning dose before breakfast; in urinary retention after surgery, 5mg daily or 500μg by intramuscular injection. It is sometimes used in neurogenic bladder disorders. Side-effects are nausea, abdominal cramp, diarrhoea and weakness.

disulfiram Tetraethylthiuram disulphide. When taken with even small amounts of alcohol, acetaldehyde accumulates in the body, with side-effects such as flushing, giddiness, vomiting and headache that may be severe. Disulfiram is used in chronic alcoholism, but prolonged treatment and co-operation of the patient are essential. *Dose:* 100–200mg daily. Acute confusion may occur if given at the same time as metronidazole.

dithranol Synthetic compound used locally in the treatment of psoriasis. The drug is a powerful irritant, and treatment should be commenced with a simple ointment or zinc paste containing 0.1%, gradually increased to 1% if well tolerated. Higher concentrations are sometimes used in 'short-contact-time' therapy.

diuretics The most widely used group of diuretics is the thiazides, represented by bendrofluazide (see page 194). They act mainly by increasing the excretion of sodium by inhibiting its reabsorption by the distal tubule of the kidney, and evoke a rapid response which may persist over 12–24 hrs, although some, such as chlorthalidone, have a still longer action. They are given in mild cardiac failure, oedema and in hypertension, but in more severe conditions, and in pulmonary oedema, the more powerful 'loop' diuretics, such as frusemide, which act at a different point, are preferred. A side-effect of some thiazides is an increase in the excretion of potassium which may require the use of potassium supplements or a change to a potassium-sparing diuretic such as triamterene. Spironolactone, an aldosterone antagonist, is a more powerful diuretic, of value in resistant oedema. Osmotic diuretics such as mannitol are used mainly in cerebral oedema. Simple diuretics such as potassium citrate, are mainly used to alkalize the urine and promote diuresis in cystitis and similar conditions.

dobutamine A sympathomimetic agent similar to isoprenaline, but with a more selective action on the beta$_1$ receptors in the heart. It increases contractility, and is less likely to cause tachycardia. Useful in acute heart failure and cardiogenic and septic shock. *Dose:* 2.5–10μg/kg/minute by intravenous infusion, carefully adjusted to need.

docusate A surface-active agent used as a faeces-softening laxative. See dioctyl sodium succinate.

domperidone An anti-emetic that functions as a dopamine antagonist, as it prevents dopamine from reaching the receptors in the chemoreceptor trigger zone (see anti-emetics). It is mainly of value in the severe nausea and vomiting caused by cytotoxic drugs, and as it also stimulates intestinal motility, it is useful in promoting the transit of barium sulphate in radiological investigations. It is of less value in post-operative and travel sickness. *Dose:* 10–20mg 4 to 8-hrly; 30–60mg by suppository. Sedative side-effects are infrequent, as domperidone does not cross the blood-brain barrier. See page 208.

dopamine A sympathomimetic agent with actions and uses similar to dobutamine. *Dose:* 2–5μg/kg/minute by slow intravenous infusion. Careful control of dose is essential, as dopamine may cause vasoconstriction with higher doses and increase the risk of heart failure. Dopamine is also a central neurotransmitter, and a deficiency is associated with parkinsonism. See levodopa and page 210.

dothiepin A tricyclic antidepressant with the uses and side-effects of amitriptyline, *q.v.* It is used in the treatment of depression when a sedative action is also indicated. *Dose:* 75–150mg daily. It may also be given as a single nightly dose to reduce daytime drowsiness.

doxapram A respiratory stimulant useful in post-operative respiratory depression, or that caused by narcotic analgesics. *Dose:* by intravenous injection 1–4.5mg/kg/min according to need. It is also given by intravenous infusion in doses controlled by arterial blood gas studies. Side-effects include hypertension, bronchospasm and tachycardia.

doxazocin An alpha-adrenoceptor blocking agent of the prazosin type, but with a longer action that permits a single daily dose. Dose in hypertension 1mg initially, slowly increased after 7–14 days to 2mg daily, up to a daily maximum of 16mg, usually in association with other antihypertensive drugs. Side-effects are dizziness and postural hypotension, and initial therapy, as with prazosin, requires care.

doxepin An antidepressant with the actions, uses and side-effects of dothiepin. *Dose:* 30–300mg daily; a single dose of 100mg is sometimes given at night.

doxorubicin A cytotoxic antibiotic widely used in leukaemia, lymphosarcoma, breast and lung cancer. *Dose:* fast intravenous infusion 60–75mg/m^2 at intervals of 3 weeks, or 20–25mg/m^2 daily for 3 days. It is also used by bladder installation (50mg in 50ml of saline solution) for superficial bladder tumours. Side-effects include bone marrow depression, cardiac damage, alopecia, buccal ulceration and nausea. Doxorubicin is a skin irritant, and should be handled with care.

doxycycline A long-acting tetracycline. *Dose:* 200mg initially, followed by 100mg as a single daily dose. In acne, a dose of 50mg daily is given for some weeks. It should be taken with adequate fluid, with the patient in a sitting or standing position.

droperidol A tranquillizer with unusual properties. It is given in severe psychotic conditions such as mania, in drug-induced nausea and vomiting and for pre-operative sedation. It is also given with fentanyl to produce a state of detachment (neuroleptanalgesia. *Dose:* 20–120mg daily; 5–10mg by injection; in cancer therapy doses of 1–3mg/hr have been given by continuous intravenous infusion. Side-effects are those of chlorpromazine and haloperidol.

drostanolone A synthetic steroid with some of the anabolic and androgenic properties of testosterone, used in the treatment of carcinoma of the breast. *Dose:* 100mg once to three times a week by intramuscular injection.

dydrogesterone An orally active progestogen that is virtually free from any oestrogenic or androgenic side-effects. It is used in amenorrhoea, functional uterine bleeding, and threatened abortion. *Dose:* 10–30mg daily, increased if breakthrough bleeding occurs.

E

econazole An antifungal agent similar in actions and uses to clotrimazole.

ecothiopate A potent and long-acting miotic that has been used in glaucoma as eye-drops of 0.03–0.25%. It may cause cataract; its availability is strictly limited.

edrophonium A very short-acting drug of the neostigmine type. It is used in the diagnosis of myasthenia gravis. *Dose:* 2–10mg by intravenous injection, which causes a marked but transient increase in muscle power if myasthenia gravis is present.

emetine An alkaloid obtained from ipecacuanha, and formerly used in the injection treatment of amoebiasis. Now replaced by metronidazole.

enalapril An ACE inhibitor used in the treatment of all types of hypertension, and in congestic heart failure, often together with a diuretic. *Dose:* 5mg daily initially, increased as required up to 40mg daily, and often given as a single dose. Dizziness, hypotension and loss of taste are some side-effects.

enflurane An inhalation anaesthetic with the actions and uses of halothane, but less potent.

enoxacin A quinolone antibacterial agent used in urinary tract, soft tissue and skin infections. *Dose:* 200–400mg daily for 7 to 14 days; in gonorrhoea a single dose of 400mg. Side-effects are those of the related ciprofloxacin, cinoxacin and nalidixic acid.

enoxaparin A heparin fraction with the general properties of heparin, yet it has little influence on blood platelet aggregation. It is given for presurgical prophylaxis in doses of 20mg by *subcutaneous* injection as a single daily dose for 7–10 days.

enoximone An inhibitor of the enzyme phosphodiesterase. It has a digoxin-like action on the myocardium and is used in congestive heart failure not responding to other drugs. *Dose:* by intravenous infusion: 90μg/kg/min initially; followed by supportive doses of 20μg/kg as required up to a maximum of 24mg/kg over 24 hrs. Side-effects are hypotension, ectopic beats and gastro-intestinal disturbances.

ephedrine A sympathomimetic agent once widely used in asthma and bronchospasm in doses of 45–120mg daily, but now largely replaced by drugs of the salbutamol type. It is sometimes useful in nocturnal enuresis, and also used as nasal drops (0.5%) to relieve nasal congestion. Side-effects are restlessness and insomnia.

epirubicin A cytotoxic agent with the actions, uses and side-effects of doxorubicin. *Dose:* 75–90mg/m^2 as free-flowing intravenous infusion repeated at intervals of 3 weeks. The side-effects and cardiotoxicity are less severe than those of doxorubicin.

epoetin beta See erythropoietin.

epoprostenol A prostaglandin present in the walls of blood vessels that inhibits platelet aggregation. It is used to preserve platelet function during cardiopulmonary bypass and charcoal haemoperfusion, and as an alternative to heparin in renal dialysis. *Dose:* 10–20 nanograms/kg/min by i.v. infusion. Smaller doses in renal dialysis. It is also a vasodilator, and side-effects are flushing and hypotension.

ergocalciferol Calciferol.

ergometrine The principal alkaloid of ergot. It promotes uterine contraction and is used for the rapid control of postpartum haemorrhage. Dangerous in the early stages of labour. *Dose:* 0.5–1mg orally; or 200–500μg by injection. Side-effects are nausea and transient hypertension.

ergot A fungus that develops in rye and replaces the normal grain. The active principles include ergometrine and ergotamine. Chronic toxic effects characterized by gangrene of the extremities, have followed the use of ergot-contaminated rye bread.

ergotamine An alkaloid of ergot that constricts the cranial arteries, and is used solely for the relief of the headache of migraine not responding to analgesic therapy. Early treatment evokes the best response. *Dose:* 2mg initially up to 6mg during an attack, not to be repeated until after an interval of some days. Total dose in one week: 10–12mg. It is also given by oral inhalation in doses of 360μg (one puff), repeated after 5 min, up to a maximum of 6 puffs daily. Side-effects include headache and nausea, and the drug should be withdrawn if tingling of the extremities occurs. Ergotamine is *not* suitable for prophylaxis because of the risks of toxicity.

erythromycin An antibiotic, resembling penicillin in its general range of activity, with the advantage of being active orally. It is useful in streptococcal and respiratory infections and in penicillin-resistant staphylococcal infections. Erythromycin is also of value in penicillin-sensitive patients. It is also given as a prophylactic before dental surgery. *Dose:* up to 4g daily; in severe infections it may be given by slow intravenous infusion. Side-effects include nausea and vomiting, and diarrhoea may occur after high doses. Care is necessary in hepatic impairment. Preparations of erythromycin *estolate* are contra-indicated in liver disease. Erythromycin may potentiate the action of warfarin.

eserine See physostigmine.

estramustine A compound of oestradiol and mustine, designed to release mustine at oestrogen-receptor sites. It has a more localized action and so causes less myelodepression. It is used mainly in prostatic carcinoma, especially when resistant to other therapy. *Dose:* 0.56–1.4g daily. Side-effects include gastrointestinal disturbances,nausea and gynaecomastia.

ethacrynic acid A loop diuretic with a rapid and intense action used mainly in oliguria due to renal failure. *Dose:* 50mg daily initially, increased as required up to a maximum of 400mg daily or on alternate days. Ethacrynic acid is also given by slow intravenous injection in doses of 50–100mg in acute or refractory conditions. Side-effects include nausea, diarrhoea and deafness. Some hypotension may occur initially.

ethambutol An antitubercular drug. *Dose:* 15mg/kg daily, together with rifampicin or isoniazid. Lower doses should be given in renal damage. It may cause visual disturbances with loss of acuity, but recovery is usually complete on withdrawal of the drug.

ethamivan A respiratory stimulant similar to nikethamide. *Dose:* 12.5–25mg orally; 100mg as required by intravenous injection.

ethamsylate A systemically effective haemostatic agent used to control bleeding from small blood vessels as in haematuria, or in surgery. *Dose:* up to 2g daily; 500mg by injection as necessary.

ethanolamine oleate A sclerosing agent used for varicose veins and bleeding oesophageal varices. *Dose:* by intravenous injection, 2–5ml.

ether A colourless inflammable liquid, once widely used as a general anaesthetic but now largely replaced by halothane.

ethinyloestradiol A widely used synthetic oestrogen more active than stilboestrol, and with fewer side-effects. Used to control menopausal symptoms, and in amenorrhoea, uterine hypoplasia, functional uterine bleeding, and other conditions where oestrogen therapy is indicated including prostatic carcinoma. *Dose:* 10–50μg daily; in carcinoma of the prostate, 1–3mg daily. Side-effects are nausea, weight gain, breast enlargement, rash and jaundice. It is present with a progestogen in many oral contraceptive products (see pp. 278–280).

ethionamide A second-line antileprotic drug given in doses of 250–375mg daily, as part of a multidrug therapy.

ethoglucid A cytotoxic agent used mainly in bladder papillomatosis. *Dose:* by instillation; 100ml of a 1% solution at weekly intervals for some months. Side-effects are frequency and dysuria.

ethosuximide An anticonvulsant for the treatment of petit mal epilepsy. May be used alone, or combined with other anticonvulsants, and it is often of value in patients not responding to other drugs. *Dose:* 500mg daily initially, gradually increased if required, to a maximum of 2g daily. Care is necessary in renal or hepatic disease.

Drowsiness, headache and gastro-intestinal disorders are some side-effects. See page 192.

ethyl chloride A volatile liquid that has been used as a local anaesthetic by virtue of the intense cold produced when sprayed on the skin.

ethynodiol A progestogen, present in some oral contraceptives (see pp. 278–280).

etidronate See disodium etidronate.

etodolac A non-steroidal anti-inflammatory agent of the naproxen type, with similar actions, uses and side-effects. *Dose:* in rheumatoid conditions, 400mg daily.

etomidate A short-acting intravenous hypnotic used for the induction of anaesthesia. It causes little cardiac disturbance or hypertension, but muscle movement and pain may occur during injection. *Dose:* 300μg/kg by intravenous injection.

etoposide A cytotoxic agent used in small-cell lung cancer and resistant testicular cancers. It is given in daily doses based on skin area for 5 days, repeated after 21 days according to response. *Dose:* 120–240mg/m^2 daily orally; by intravenous infusion 60–120mg/m^2, and care must be taken to avoid extravasation. Side-effects include nausea, alopecia and myelosuppression.

etretinate A potent derivative of vitamin A, used in the treatment of severe psoriasis. Its use requires careful and continued control. *Dose:* 0.25–1mg/kg daily. The response to treatment may be slow in onset, and therapy for some weeks is usually required. Side-effects include dryness of the mouth, alopecia, pruritus and nose-bleeding.

eusol A chlorine antiseptic solution used as lotion, or as compress. The solution should be freshly prepared.

evening primrose oil See gamolenic acid.

eye-drops Weak solutions of drugs for the treatment of ocular conditions. They may be antibacterial, antifungal or antiviral in action, or may be used for non-infective conditions such as glaucoma, or for diagnosis. For routine use they are supplied sterile in multiple-application containers, but are intended for individual use only. They contain preservatives, but may be used for up to one month after the container has been opened. In eye-surgery, single application products are preferred. Occasionally, enough of a drug may be absorbed from eye-drops to have systemic effects, and corticosteroids, if used as eye-drops over a prolonged period, may cause 'steroid glaucoma'. Care should be taken with contact lenses, and ideally they should not be worn during eye-drop treatment. Soft contact lenses can absorb the preservatives, which may cause irritation.

F

famotidine An H_2-receptor antagonist with the uses and side-effects of cimetidine, but a longer action. Dose in benign peptic ulcer: 40mg at night for 4–8 weeks; 20mg at night for the prevention of recurrence. In Zollinger-Ellison syndrome, doses of 20mg 6-hrly are given. See page 212.

Fansidar Pyrimethamine, 25mg with sulfadoxine, 500mg. Both these drugs block the formation of folinic acid in the malarial parasite, but the combination is more effective. Of value in patients unable to tolerate chloroquine, and in chloroquine-resistant malaria. *Dose:* for treatment, two or three tablets as a single dose, not to be repeated for at least 7 days. (Fansidar is no longer recommended for prophylaxis, as fatalities have followed such use).

felodipine A calcium antagonist used in the treatment of hypertension generally (see calcium channel blocking agents). *Dose:* 5mg daily initially, adjusted to maintenance doses up to 10mg daily. Tablets should be taken in the morning, and swallowed whole with water. No adjustment of dose necessary for elderly patients, but care is required in marked hepatic impairment. Hypotension with tachycardia may occur with susceptible patients.

felypressin A vasopressin derivative, used as a vasoconstrictor in local anaesthetic solutions for dental use, when sympathetic pressor drugs are contra-indicated.

fenbufen A non-steroidal anti-inflammatory agent used for the relief of pain and inflammation in rheumatoid arthritis and similar conditions. *Dose:* 600–900mg daily. Like related drugs, it may cause gastro-intestinal disturbance and dizziness, but the incidence of rash is more frequent and requires withdrawal of the drug.

fencamfamin A weak CNS stimulant, present in some preparations given for fatigue and debility.

fenfluramine An appetite depressant without the stimulant effects of related drugs. It is used in the treatment of obesity. *Dose:* 60–120mg daily. Side-effects are sedation, dizziness and gastro-intestinal disturbances.

fenofibrate A plasma lipid-regulating agent of the clofibrate type, with similar uses and side-effects. *Dose:* 300mg initially, with food, later 200–400mg daily according to need. See page 197.

fenoprofen A non-steroidal anti-inflammatory and anti-rheumatic agent. It is also used as a mild analgesic in a variety of painful conditions. *Dose:* 900mg–3g daily. Side-effects include nausea, dizziness, vertigo and rash.

fenoterol A sympathomimetic agent with the actions, uses and side-effects of salbutamol. Dose by oral inhalation 200–400mg (1–2 puffs) up to four times a day.

fentanyl A narcotic analgesic, used mainly in thiopentone anaesthesia to increase the response and permit a reduction in dose of thiopentone, especially in poor-risk patients. It is also used with droperidol, to produce a state of neuroleptanalgesia. *Dose:* 50–200μg by intravenous injection.

ferrous sulphate, fumerate, gluconate and succinate These iron salts are used in the prophylaxis and treatment of iron-deficiency anaemias. Ferrous sulphate is the standard drug, given in doses of 600mg daily, but it may cause gastric disturbance in some patients, and ferrous fumarate, gluconate and succinate are better tolerated alternatives. Some better tolerated slow-release products are available, but may be less well absorbed. Ferrous sulphate tablets are potentially dangerous for small children, and death has occurred after accidental administration. See desferrioxamine.

fibrinolytic agents Drugs used to break up blood clots, and so are of value in thrombosis. See alteplase, anistreplase, streptokinase and urokinase.

filgrastim Filgrastim, like erythropoetin, is one of a group of natural growth factors concerned with bone marrow activity. It stimulates the development of neutrophils, the production of which is depressed during cytotoxic therapy. The neutropenia thus caused increases the risks of infection, but the neutrophil count can be restored by filgrastim. It is used mainly in the neutropenia associated with the cytotoxic treatment of non-myeloid malignancy. *Dose:* 5μg/kg daily by subcutaneous injection or intravenous infusion for 14 days, or until the neutrophil count returns to normal. The first dose should be given at least 24 hrs after chemotherapy. Following cessation of filgrastim treatment, there is usually a 50% reduction in the neutrophil count within 2 days. The main side-effects are musculoskeletal pain and dysuria.

flavoxate An antispasmodic of value in urinary disorders such as dysuria, frequency and related conditions. *Dose:* 600mg daily. Side-effects include dry mouth and blurred vision. Care is necessary in glaucoma.

flecainide An orally active anti-arrhythmic agent of the lignocaine type. It chiefly influences conduction in the bundle of His, and is of value in serious ventricular tachycardia and extrasystoles. *Dose:* 200–400mg daily. May be given by slow intravenous injection in doses of 2mg/kg in acute conditions. Care is necessary in patients with pacemakers, and in renal impairment. Dizziness and visual disturbances are side-effects.

fluclorolone A highly potent locally acting corticosteroid used as cream and ointment (0.025%) in severely inflamed skin disorders not responding to other therapy.

flucloxacillin A derivative of cloxacillin, that is absorbed more readily when given orally. It is used mainly in infections due to penicillinase-producing penicillin-resistant staphylococci. *Dose:* 1g daily before food; by injection 1–4g daily, but larger doses are given in very severe infections. Side-effects are those of the penicillins generally. See co-fluampicil.

fluconazole A local and systemically acting synthetic antifungal agent. *Dose:* in oral candidiasis 50mg daily for 7–14 days: in vaginal candidiasis a single dose of 150mg. Dose in systemic candidiasis and cryptococcosis 200–400mg daily orally or by intravenous infusion. Side-effects include nausea and abdominal discomfort.

flucytosine A synthetic antifungal agent used in systemic yeast infections such as candidiasis and cryptococcosis. *Dose:* orally or intravenously, 100–200mg/kg daily. It may cause some bone marrow deprèssion, and sensitivity tests should be carried out before and during treatment, as resistance to the drug may limit its value. Care is necessary in renal and hepatic impairment. Side-effects include nausea, diarrhoea and rash.

fludrocortisone A synthetic steroid with a very powerful salt-retaining action. Valuable in adrenal deficiency states such as Addison's disease to supplement hydrocortisone treatment. *Dose:* 50–300μg daily. The side-effects are those common to the corticosteroids in general.

flumazenil A benzodiazepine antagonist used in anaesthesia to reverse the sedative effects of benzodiazepines. *Dose:* 200μg initally by intravenous injection, with subsequent doses of 100μg at 1 min intervals, up to a maximum of 1mg. Further doses may be given by intravenous infusion if drowsiness returns, as the action of flumazenil is short.

flunisolide A potent corticosteroid used locally in the more severe forms of hay-fever and other nasal allergies. *Dose:* by nasal inhalation, 50μg (two sprays), two or three times a day, continued for 2–3 weeks, or longer if required.

flunitrazepam A benzodiazepine with an hypnotic action and used for the short-term treatment of insomnia. *Dose:* 0.5–1mg. Side-effects include drowsiness, ataxia and visual disturbances.

fluocinolone A topically active corticosteroid. Used as cream, ointment or lotion (0.0025–0.025%) in severe, inflamed, corticosteroid-responsive skin disorders. Excessive application should be avoided.

fluocinonide A locally effective anti-inflammatory steroid similar to fluocinolone.

fluocortolone A potent, locally acting corticosteroid used as cream or ointment (0.025%) in severe, inflamed skin conditions.

fluorescein An orange-red dye; solutions have a strong green fluorescence. Used as eye-drops (2%) for detecting corneal lesions, as areas of cornea denuded of epithelium stain green. Sometimes given by injection to facilitate examination of retinal blood vessels. Fluorescein dilaurate is given orally in a dose of 350mg as a test of pancreatic function.

fluorometholone A corticosteroid used as eye-drops (0.1%) for inflammatory conditions of the eye.

fluorouracil A cytotoxic agent used in the palliative treatment of carcinoma of the breast and gastrointestinal tract and other solid tumours. *Dose:* 15mg/kg orally daily for 6 days, then once weekly; or by 15mg/kg intravenous infusion, weekly up to a total dose of 12–15g. Side-effects include alopecia, and dermatitis, but haematotoxicity, severe gastrointestinal disturbance and haemorrhage may limit treatment. Fluorouracil is used locally as a cream (5%) in malignant skin lesions.

Fluosol An emulsion of fluohydrocarbons used as an oxygen-carrying blood substitute in coronary angioplasty as an alternative to bypass surgery. The product is supplied frozen, and is reconstituted before use.

fluoxetine An antidepressant that acts by selectively inhibiting the uptake of serotonin. Dose in depression 20mg daily. Side-effects are gastro-intestinal disturbances, dizziness and anorexia; rash is an indication of withdrawal. It should not be used with other drugs that influence serotonin uptake.

flupenthixol A tranquillizer similar to fluphenazine, and used in the treatment of schizophrenia, especially with apathy and withdrawal. It also has an antidepressant action. *Dose:* 6–8mg daily initially, with subsequent adjustment according to need. It may cause some restlessness and insomnia. Dose by deep intramuscular injection, 20–40mg every 2–4 weeks. Dose in depression: 500μg–3mg daily. The side-effects are similar to those of chlorpromazine.

fluphenazine An antipsychotic drug with the actions and uses of chlorpromazine, but with reduced sedative and anticholinergic side-effects, although extrapyramidal symptoms may be increased. *Dose:* 2–10mg initially in schizophrenia adjusted up to 20mg daily. In severe anxiety states 1–4mg. For depot treatment, 12.5–100mg of the decanoate by deep intramuscular injection every 12–14 days according to response.

flurandrenolone A potent locally acting corticosteroid used as a cream or ointment (0.0125%–0.05%) in severe skin disorders not responding to other therapy.

flurazepam A benzodiazepine hypnotic for the short-term treatment of insomnia. *Dose:* 15–30mg nightly. It may cause daytime sedation in some patients.

flurbiprofen A non-steroid anti-inflammatory drug with the actions, uses and side-effects of naproxen. It is used in the relief of pain and inflammation in rheumatoid and arthritic conditions, and in other musculoskeletal disorders. *Dose:* 150mg daily, after food, increased up to 300mg daily if necessary. Suppositories of 100mg are available. Care is necessary in peptic ulcer, and in aspirin-sensitive asthmatic patients.

fluspirilene A potent antipsychotic drug, used for the maintenance control of schizophrenia and related psychoses. *Dose:* by deep intramuscular injection, 2mg weekly, adjusted up to 20mg weekly. It is less sedating and with fewer extrapyramidal side-effects than other chlorpromazine-like drugs.

flutamide Flutamide is an androgen blocking agent, and inhibits the action of androgens on target organs. It is used in advanced prostatic cancer not responding to other drugs, usually in association with goserilin or related substances. *Dose:* 750mg daily. Side-effects include gynaecomastia. Liver function should be checked, and dosage of anticoagulants may need adjustment.

fluticasone A topical corticosteroid of increased potency. Used as a metered dose pump for the prophylaxis and treatment of seasonal allergic rhinitis and hay fever. *Dose:* 50μg (two sprays) into each nostril once a day in the morning. Maximum relief may not be obtained for 3–4 days. Systemic absorption extremely low.

fluvoxamine An antidepressant that appears to act by inhibiting the central re-uptake of serotonin. It is used mainly for maintenance treatment during depressive illness. *Dose:* 100–300mg daily; a steady plasma level is normally reached within 10–14 days. Side-effects after initial nausea may include somnolence, constipation and agitation. It should not be used with other drugs that increase serotonin uptake. Fluvoxamine may increase the plasma levels of propranolol and warfarin.

folic acid A constituent of the vitamin B group. It is essential for cell division and the growth and development of normal red blood cells. The main therapeutic use is in the treatment of megaloblastic anaemias due to folic acid deficiency. *Dose:* 15mg daily initially; 5mg weekly may be adequate after the haematological response has been obtained. Sometimes given with anti-epileptic drugs, as long-term therapy may cause a folic acid deficiency. Small doses are present in many iron preparations to prevent the megaloblastic anaemia that may occur in later stages of pregnancy. It must not be used alone in pernicious anaemia, as it cannot prevent the degeneration of the central nervous system associated with that disease.

folinic acid A methotrexate antidote. It is given at the end of a course of methotrexate to reduce the toxic effects on normal cells and in methotrexate-overdose, the so-called Leucovorin Rescue treatment. *Dose:* up to 120mg over 24 hrs by intramuscular injection (or intravenously), with 15mg orally for another 48 hrs.

formaldehyde A powerful but toxic germicide used mainly as 'formalin' in the disinfection of rooms, and as 'formol-saline' (5% in normal saline) for the preservation of pathological specimens. Warts have been treated with a 3% solution.

formalin A 40% solution of formaldehyde.

foscarnet An antiviral agent for the treatment of sight-damaging cytomegalovirus retinitis in AIDS patients as an alternative to ganciclovir. *Dose:* 20μg/kg by continuous intravenous infusion, with subsequent infusion at a rate dependent on renal function.

fosfestrol A water-soluble derivative of stilboestrol. It is metabolized by the enzyme acid phosphatase to liberate stilboestrol in tissues rich in that enzyme, and so it is of value in prostatic carcinoma. *Dose:* 300–600mg daily, adjusted as required. Dose by slow intravenous injection, 552–1104mg daily for 5 days or more. Maintenance dose: 276mg i.v. once or twice a week. Perineal pain is a side-effect.

fosinopril An ACE inhibitor indicated in hypertension when standard therapy is ineffective or unsuitable. *Dose:* 10mg daily initially, adjusted after 4 weeks up to 40mg according to need. It is eliminated by the liver as well as the kidneys, and may have some advantages in renal impairment. See ACE inhibitors.

framycetin An antibiotic resembling neomycin in general properties. Used as cream, ointment and lotion (0.3–0.5%). Given by subconjunctival injection in eye infections.

French chalk Talc.

friar's balsam Contains benzoin, storax, aloes, balsam of tolu. Official name Compound Tincture of Benzoin. (See benzoin.)

frusemide A loop diuretic with a powerful and intense action of short duration. Often effective in conditions no longer responding to thiazide diuretics. *Dose:* 20–80mg daily or on alternate days, or 20–50mg i.m. or i.v. Much larger oral doses, varying from 250mg up to a single maximum dose of 2g may be required in renal failure and oliguria. Side-effects include nausea, diarrhoea and cramp. Supplementary potassium is usually necessary as with other powerful diuretics.

fusidic acid Sodium fusidate.

G

gallamine A synthetic non-depolarizing (competitive) muscle relaxant with an action similar to that of tubocurarine, but the effect is more rapid and less prolonged. It is used extensively in surgery as it is well tolerated although some tachycardia may occur. *Dose:* 80–120mg initially intravenously with small subsequent doses according to need and response. The action of the drug may be terminated, as with tubocurarine, by the injection of neostigmine, 2.5–5mg, together with atropine, 0.5–1mg.

gamolinic acid A derivative of linoleic acid present in evening primrose oil. It is said to be of value in atopic eczema. *Dose:* 320–480mg daily. It is also used in mastalgia (breast pain) in doses of 240–320mg daily, but the response is slow (8–12 weeks).

gammaglobulin Immunoglobulin.

ganciclovir An antiviral agent similar to acyclovir, but more toxic. It is used only in sight- and life-threatening infections with cytomegalovirus (CMV) in immunocompromised patients. Dose by intravenous infusion 5mg/kg every 12 hours for 14–21 days, with maintenance doses of 5mg/kg daily. The solution is very alkaline, and injection requires care. Regular blood counts are essential.

Gee's linctus A soothing cough linctus containing camphorated tincture of opium, oxymel of squill and syrup of tolu. *Dose:* 2–4ml.

gelatin A protein obtained by the hydrolysis of animal tissues. Used orally as nutrient jellies, and specially refined solutions have been used as blood volume expanders (see dextran). Absorbable gelatin sponge is used as a haemostat.

gemeprost A synthetic prostaglandin used to dilate the cervix uteri in first trimester abortion. *Dose:* 1mg as a pessary 3 hours before surgery. Side-effects are mild uterine pain and vaginal bleeding initially; nausea and diarrhoea are later effects.

gemfibrozil A plasma lipid regulating agent, with the actions and uses of bezafibrate and clofibrate. *Dose:* 900mg–1.5mg daily, with regular checks on plasma lipid levels. Treatment should be withdrawn after 3 months if the response is unsatisfactory. Gemfibrozil may potentiate the action of oral anticoagulants, the dose of which should be adjusted. Side-effects include nausea, diarrhoea, abdominal pain, rash and dizziness. See page 197.

gentamicin An aminoglycoside antibiotic, active against a wide range of Gram-negative organisms, including *Pseudomonas aeruginosa*, as well as against many Gram-positive bacteria, although it is not very active against anaerobic organisms. It is of great value in septicaemia and meningitis, as well as in bacterial endocarditis. *Dose:* 2–5mg/kg daily by intramuscular injection or intravenous infusion. In serious or undiagnosed infections, supplementary treatment with a penicillin or metronidazole may be required. In common with other aminoglycosides, gentamicin has ototoxic and nephrotoxic side-effects, and dosage requires care when renal function is inadequate, and also in elderly patients. Gentamicin is also used locally as cream or ointment (0.3%) and as eye-drops (0.3%).

gentian violet Crystal violet.

gestrinone An antiprogestogen used in endometriosis that appears to act indirectly by suppressing gonadotrophin production. *Dose:* 2.5mg twice weekly on the same days each week for 6 months. Side-effects are fluid retention, acne and voice changes.

gestronol A synthetic progestogen used in the treatment of endometrial carcinoma and benign prostatic hypertrophy. *Dose:* 200–400mg i.m. once a week.

glibenclamide An orally active hypoglycaemic agent similar to chlorpropamide. *Dose:* 5–15mg daily, according to need and response.

gliclazide A sulphonylurea with the actions and uses of chlorpropamide and related drugs. *Dose:* 40–320mg orally.

glipizide A sulphonylurea, used like chlorpropamide in diabetes, but effective in much lower doses. *Dose:* 5mg initially, maintenance, 2.5–40mg daily.

gliquidone An oral hypoglycaemic agent similar to chlorpropamide. Effective in maturity-onset diabetes. *Dose:* 40–60mg daily, but up to 180mg daily have been given.

glucagon A hormone of the alpha cells of the pancreas which raises the blood sugar level by mobilizing liver glycogen. Used in acute hypoglycaemia. *Dose:* 0.5–1mg by subcutaneous, intramuscular or intravenous injection, repeated in 20 minutes if necessary.

glucocorticoids Those corticosteroids with an anti-inflammatory action similar to hydrocortisone, as distinct from the mineralocorticoids, such as fludrocortisone, used in Addison's disease. They differ in anti-inflammatory potency, and 0.75mg of dexamethasone is considered equivalent to 20mg of hydrocortisone. See Table 31.

glucose Also known as dextrose. A readily absorbed carbohydrate present in many sweet fruits, but obtained commercially by the hydrolysis of starch. It is given orally as a dietary supplement; in acidosis, and to raise the glycogen reserves of the liver in hepatic damage. Given by intravenous infusion as a 5% solution, or as a glucose-saline infusion in dehydration and shock, and after surgery until fluids can be taken by mouth.

glutaraldehyde A disinfectant of the formaldehyde type, but with a more rapid and powerful action. Effective against a wide range of organisms, including viruses. Used mainly for instrument sterilization as a 2% solution. Usually activated before use by the addition of a corrosion inhibitor. Such activated solutions are stable for about 2 weeks. It is also used as a 10% solution for the removal of plantar warts.

glycerin, glycerol A clear syrupy liquid used as a sweetening agent in mixtures and linctuses. It promotes drainage when applied to inflamed areas, and is used as a paste with magnesium sulphate for boils. It is frequently used in the form of suppositories for constipation. *Dose:* 1–1.5g/kg orally in glaucoma and before cataract surgery to lower the intra-ocular pressure.

glyceryl trinitrate A powerful but short-acting vasodilator. It is used mainly in the control of angina pectoris. *Dose:* 300, 500 or 600μg tablets which should be dissolved under the tongue for a rapid response. An aerosol spray (400μg per dose), as well as long-acting tablets are also available. Tolerance may occur with prolonged therapy. Side-effects are a throbbing headache, flushing and tachycardia. It is also used locally for an extended action as ointment and medicated patches. Also given by intravenous infusion to control hypertension and ischaemia during cardiovascular surgery and in left ventricular failure. *Dose:* 10–200μg/minute in dextrose-saline.

glycopyrronium A synthetic atropine-like antispasmodic used for pre-operative medication in doses of 200–400mg by intramuscular or intravenous injection. It has the side-effects of anticholinergic drugs such as dryness of the mouth and blurred vision. Contra-indicated in glaucoma.

gold therapy See sodium aurothiomalate.

gonadorelin The gonadotrophin-releasing hormone of the hypothalamus. It is used to assess pituitary function, as doses of 100μg by intravenous injection normally lead to a rapid rise in the plasma level of the luteinizing and follicle-stimulating hormones. In amenorrhoea and infertility due to gonadorelin insufficiency, it is given by pulsed subcutaneous infusion in doses of 10–20μg every 90 minutes, day and night. Treatment for up to 6 months may be required. Side-effects are uncommon.

goserelin A highly potent, synthetic analogue of the hypothalamic hormone LHRH. It suppresses the production of testosterone, and is used in the treatment of hormone-dependent carcinoma of the prostate. *Dose:* 3.6mg by subcutaneous injection every 28 days. Side-effects include impotence, hot flushes, rash and breast swelling and tenderness. A transient rise in the serum testosterone level and in bone pain may occur initially.

gramicidin A mixture of antibiotics effective against many Gram-positive organisms, but it is too toxic for systemic use. Used topically in infected skin conditions, usually in association with neomycin and hydrocortisone.

granisetron A serotonin (5-HT) antagonist with a highly selective and powerful anti-emetic action mediated by its effects on the $5\text{-}HT_3$ receptors. It is used in the prevention and treatment of the severe nausea and vomiting induced by potent cytotoxic drugs such as cisplatin. It is given by intravenous infusion in doses of 3mg, which give rapid relief that may extend over 24 hrs. Further doses if required may be given up to a maximum of 9mg daily. For prophylaxis, a dose of 3mg should be given before chemotherapy is commenced. Headache and constipation are common side-effects, but central disturbances such as extra-pyramidal symptoms are unlikely to occur.

griseofulvin An orally effective but slow-acting antifungal antibiotic that is deposited selectively in the skin, hair and nails. It is used in the systemic treatment of ringworm and other dermatophyte infections of the keratin-containing tissues, but only when other treatment has failed. *Dose:* 0.5–1g daily, but prolonged therapy is required. Side-effects are headache, nausea, rash and photosensitivity. It may also reduce the effects of oral contraceptives.

growth hormone See somatotropin.

guanethidine An anti-hypertensive drug that brings about a reduction in blood pressure by blocking transmission in adrenergic nerves, and preventing the release of noradrenaline. It has been used in the treatment of all types of hypertension, often with a thiazide diuretic, but its value has declined, as it may cause postural hypotension. It remains useful as part of combined therapy in resistant hypertension *Dose:* 20mg daily, increased by 10mg at weekly intervals according to response, up to 100mg daily, although sometimes larger doses are required. Dose by intramuscular injection, 10–

20mg as required. Diarrhoea, weakness, nasal congestion and bradycardia are common side-effects. Guanethidine is occasionally used as eye-drops (1–5%) in glaucoma and thyrotoxicosis.

guar gum A vegetable gum that, when taken with food, appears to retard the absorption of glucose. It is sometimes used in the supplementary treatment of diabetes mellitus. *Dose:* up to 15g daily, usually sprinkled on food. It is essential that a dose should be taken with an adequate fluid intake, and that the final dose is not taken at bedtime. Side-effects are flatulence and abdominal distension.

H

HA-1A See human monoclonal IgM antibody.

halcinonide A locally effective corticosteroid used in severe inflammatory skin conditions not responding to other corticosteroids. It is applied sparingly as a 0.1% cream.

halibut-liver oil A rich source of vitamins A and D. *Dose:* 0.2–0.5ml.

halofantrine An antimalarial, acting at the erythrocytic stage of the life cycle of Plasmodium, and useful in chloroquine or multi-drug resistant malaria. *Dose:* 500mg 6-hrly for three doses. Side-effects are nausea, vomiting and diarrhoea. Contra-indicated in pregnancy.

haloperidol A tranquillizer chemically unrelated to chlorpromazine, but having a basically similar but longer action. Valuable in mania and schizophrenic excitement. *Dose:* 5–20mg daily, up to a maximum of 200mg, reduced later according to response. By i.m. injection for rapid control of hyperactive psychotic patients, 5–30mg initially followed by 5mg as required. For depot treatment, it is given as haloperidol decanoate, 50–300mg by deep i.m. injection every 4 weeks. It is also given orally in doses of 500μg twice daily in severe anxiety. Doses of 1.5mg have been given for intractable hiccup. Care is necessary in liver disease. It has reduced anticholinergic and sedative side-effects, but the incidence of extra-pyramidal symptoms may be a limiting factor.

halothane A widely used non-inflammable inhalation anaesthetic, more powerful and less irritant than ether. It suppresses mucous and bronchial secretions, and reduces capillary bleeding. It has some muscle-relaxant properties, but in major surgery, supplementary treatment with a muscle relaxant such as tubarine is necessary. Halothane may cause some cardiac irregularities, but an occasional serious side-effect is a marked disturbance of liver function, particularly after further exposure to the drug within periods of 4–6 weeks. Such susceptibility cannot yet be detected, so great care is necessary in any cases of liver dysfunction.

hamamelis An extract of hamamelis or witch hazel leaves is used as an astringent in suppositories for the symptomatic relief of haemorrhoids. A distillate referred to as hamamelis or witch hazel water, is used as a soothing application for bruises and sprains.

Hartmann's solution An electrolyte-replacement solution containing sodium lactate, sodium chloride, potassium chloride, and calcium chloride; given orally or intravenously in acidosis and gastro-enteritis.

heparin The natural anticoagulant obtained from lung and liver tissue. It is widely used in the prophylaxis and treatment of deep-vein thrombosis and disseminated intravascular coagulation. *Dose:* by intravenous injection 5000 units initially, followed by 10 000 units 6-hrly according to need under laboratory control. It is sometimes given by continuous intravenous infusion. Overdosage can be controlled by the intravenous injection of protamine sulphate. Treatment with heparin may be combined with that of oral anticoagulants such as phenindione or warfarin to provide immediate action before the slow-acting oral drugs begin to take effect. Occasional side-effects include hypersensitivity reactions and alopecia. (Heparinized saline solutions are used to flush catheters and cannulas to maintain patency.)

hepatitis B vaccine A preparation of inactivated hepatitis B virus antigen for the protection of individuals highly exposed to the infection. *Dose:* 1ml by i.m. injection, repeated after 1 month and again after 6 months, as development of immunity is slow.

†**heroin** Diamorphine.

hetastarch A soluble, modified, starch that is used as a 6% solution with 0.9% sodium chloride as a plasma volume expander. *Dose:* 500–1500ml daily by i.v. infusion, up to a maximum of 20ml/kg daily. It is excreted by the kidneys, and care must be taken to avoid circulatory overload. Not for use in congestive heart failure or renal insufficiency. Side-effects are vomiting, chills, fever and urticaria.

hexachlorophane A slow-acting antiseptic used for skin sterilization, and present in some medicated soaps.

hexamine A formaldehyde derivative of low toxicity, occasionally used as a urinary antiseptic. *Dose:* 2g daily. It is usually given as hexamine hippurate to ensure acidification of the urine, without which hexamine is inactive.

histamine A compound present in a bound form in all mammalian tissues; its release is probably the ultimate cause of many allergic conditions.

histamine H_1-receptor antagonists See antihistamines.

histamine H_2-receptor antagonists Drugs that differ from conventional antihistamines in having a selective blocking action on receptors in the gastric cells that secrete acid. They are widely used in the treatment of peptic ulcer and other conditions requiring a reduction in gastric acid secretion. See cimetidine, famotidine, nizatidine, ranitidine and the proton pump inhibitor omeprazole, and page 212.

homatropine An atropine derivative with a similar but more rapid mydriatic action (15–30 minutes), but a shorter duration of effect of about 24 hrs. Eye-drops (1–2%) sometimes with cocaine.

human monoclonal IgM antibody (HA-1A) It binds with the lipid A fragment of bacterial endotoxin. In the circulation, lipid A causes necrosis leading to multiple organ failure, but its action can be inhibited by HA-1A. It is used in Gram-negative bacteraemia and septic shock, and is given as a *single* dose of 100mg by intravenous infusion as soon as possible. Transient flushing, local urticaria and hypotension are occasional side-effects.

hyaluronidase A 'spreading' factor derived from testes, and used to increase the absorption of large-volume subcutaneous injections. The injection of 1500 units of hyaluronidase, either into the injection site or mixed with the injection fluid, will promote the absorption of 500–1000mL of electrolyte solution by *subcutaneous* drip infusion.

hydralazine A vasodilator that is useful in the supplementary treatment of hypertension, but when used alone it tends to cause tachycardia and fluid retention. *Dose:* 50–100mg daily, usually with a thiazide diuretic or a beta-blocking agent. Also given in hypertensive crisis by *slow* intravenous injection in doses of 5–20mg; over-rapid injection may cause a marked fall in blood pressure. Side-effects are nausea, tachycardia and fluid retention (less likely with low doses), but a lupus erythematosus-like syndrome may occur with extended high-dose therapy.

hydrochlorothiazide A thiazide diuretic that brings about a marked increase in the excretion of salts and water, and is of value in congestive heart failure and other oedematous conditions. It is also of value in hypertension, as it reduces peripheral resistance, and potentiates the action of some other antihypertensive drugs. *Dose:* 50–100mg daily initially in oedema; maintenance, 25–50mg daily or on alternate days. In hypertension, 25–100mg daily according to need. Hydrochlorothiazide, like other thiazides, increases the excretion of potassium as well as sodium, and in extended treatment supplementary treatment with potassium chloride or effervescent potassium tablets may be required. Side-effects include nausea, rash, dizziness and photosensitivity.

hydrocortisone The principal corticosteroid, also known as cortisol, that is secreted by the adrenal cortex. It plays a major role in the metabolism of glucose, protein and calcium; in maintaining the electrolyte metabolism, and in reducing inflammatory and allergic responses. It is used in all cases of adrenocortical insufficiency, including Addison's disease and after adrenalectomy. It is also used in anaphylactic shock and asthma. It is also useful in rheumatoid disease and allergic states. It is valuable in acute lymphoblastic leukaemia and some lymphomas. In common with some other corticosteroids, hydrocortisone inhibits organ-transplant rejection, and in high doses it is given to control incipient rejection. *Dose:* varies considerably according to need: for replacement therapy, 20–30mg daily; in shock, 100–300mg or more by slow i.v. injection, repeated as required; by intra-articular injection, 5–50mg. Side-effects are numerous and include hypertension, oedema, mental disturbances, re-activation of peptic ulcer, muscle weakness and diabetes. Cushing's syndrome may occur with high doses. Hydrocortisone, unlike cortisone, is active topically, and is used as eye-drops 0.5% (usually with an antibiotic), ointment and cream (0.5% and 1%), often with an antibiotic to control any secondary infection.

hydroflumethiazide A thiazide diuretic with the actions, uses and side-effects of bendrofluazide. *Dose:* 25–100mg daily, 25–50mg daily in hypertension. See page 194.

hydrogen peroxide solution It contains 5–7% of H_2O_2, equivalent to about 20 volumes of oxygen. It has antiseptic and deodorizing properties, and is used mainly for cleaning wounds. It is also used as a mouthwash (diluted 1:7), and as ear-drops (1:4 in water or 50% alcohol).

hydrotalcite Aluminium magnesium hydroxide carbonate. An antacid said to lower the acidity of the gastric secretions to between pH3 and pH5 for over 2 hours. *Dose:* 1g as required.

hydroxocobalamin A derivative of cyanocobalamin, with similar actions and now the preferred form of vitamin B_{12} as it has a more prolonged action. *Dose:* in pernicious anaemia and other vitamin B_{12} deficiency states, 1mg initially i.m. repeated five times at intervals of 2–3 days; maintenance, 1mg by injection every 3 months. It is also given prophylactically after total gastrectomy.

hydroxyapatite A natural substance with a mineral composition somewhat similar to that of bone. It is used as a source of calcium and phosphorus in deficiency states and as a dietary supplement. Tablets of 830mg are available.

hydroxychloroquine An antimalarial with the actions, uses and side-effects of chloroquine. It is sometimes useful in rheumatoid arthritis in doses of 200–400mg daily, and in lupus erythematosus in doses of 200–400mg weekly, but side-effects are numerous, and treatment requires expert supervision.

5-hydroxytryptamine See serotonin.

hydroxyurea A cytotoxic agent sometimes used in chronic myeloid leukaemia. *Dose:* 20–30mg/kg as a single dose daily, or 80mg/kg every third day. Side-effects are nausea, skin reactions and myelosuppression.

hydroxyzine A mild tranquillizer with some sedative and antihistaminic properties. It is given in anxiety and agitation, and also in dermatoses complicated by emotional tension. *Dose:* 50–400mg daily. It has the side-effects of the antihistamines, and is not recommended in conditions where some degree of sedation is undesirable.

hyoscine Also known as scopolamine. An alkaloid obtained from plants of the belladonna group. It is a powerful hypnotic and is widely used together with papaveretum for premedication before operation. It has some antiemetic properties, and is useful in travel sickness and vertigo. *Dose:* 1.2–2.4mg daily, orally or by injection. The side-effects of mouth dryness and dizziness are those of the anticholinergic drugs generally. It is contra-indicated in glaucoma.

hyoscine butylbromide A derivative of hyoscine that differs in lacking any action on the central nervous system. It is given in spasm and hypermotility of the gastrointestinal tract, and may be useful in spasmodic dysmenorrhoea. *Dose:* 40–80mg daily; in acute spasm, 20mg by injection.

hypochlorite solutions See sodium hypochlorite.

hypromellose A cellulose-derivative that dissolves in water to form a viscid, colloidal solution. Such a solution is used as a base for eye-drops to extend the action of a dissolved ophthalmic drug; to lubricate contact lenses; and to act as a lubricant in chronic, sore eye conditions.

I

ibuprofen A non-steroidal anti-inflammatory agent widely used in rheumatoid and arthritic conditions. It is also given as an analgesic for mild to moderate pain, but it is not recommended for acute gout. *Dose:* 1.8g daily initially; maintenance dose, 600mg–1.2g daily. Care is necessary in peptic ulcer, asthma and liver dysfunction. Side-effects include gastro-intestinal disturbances, rash, headache and tinnitus. A 5% cream is available for local use.

ichthammol A thick, dark brown liquid wiuh a characteristic odour, derived from certain bituminous oils. It is a mild antiseptic and is used mainly in chronic eczema as a 10% ointment, and as solution (10%) in glycerin for ulcers and inflamed areas.

idoxuridine An antiviral agent used locally in dendritic ulcers of the eye as drops of 0.1% solution to be used every hour, or 0.5% ointment 4-hrly. A 0.1% solution is also used as a paint for oral herpetic lesions. It is also applied locally as a 5% solution in dimethyl sulphoxide in herpes zoster skin infections. It has also been used intravenously for systemic viral infections, but its toxicity limits its value. See page 196.

ifosfamide A derivative of cyclophosphamide with similar actions and uses. It is effective in lung, ovary, breast and soft-tissue tumours, as well as some malignant lymphomas. *Dose:* by intravenous infusion as a 5-day course up to a total of 8–10g/m^2, with subsequent doses at intervals of 2–4 weeks, but other dosage schemes are also in use. As with cyclophosphamide, ifosfamide must be given with mesna to reduce its urothelial toxicity.

imipenem A new antibiotic with a range of activity that includes Gram-positive and Gram-negative bacteria, as well as aerobes and anaerobes, and is indicated in infections due to such organisms. It is inactive orally, and is given by intravenous infusion in doses of 1–2g daily. As it is inactivated to some extent by kidney enzymes, it is always given together with the specific enzyme inhibitor cilastatin. The side-effects are numerous and include those common to other antibiotics, and care is necessary in hypersensitivity to the penicillins, cephalosporins and related antibiotics, and in epilepsy.

imipramine A tricyclic antidepressant with the general action, uses and side-effects of amitriptyline, but with a reduced sedative action. It has been widely used in acute endogenous depression, although the initial response may be slow, and long treatment may be required. *Dose:* 75mg daily, increased up to 200mg, with a dose of 150mg at night. It is sometimes used in the treatment of enuresis in doses of 25–50mg. Imipramine should not be given in association with or soon after monoamine oxidase inhibitors, as the effects of both drugs may be increased. Imipramine may also reduce the response to some antihypertensive drugs. See page 185.

immunoglobulin The normal product obtained from plasma is given for protection against infectious hepatitis, measles, rubella and hepatitis A in susceptible patients. More specific products are hepatitis B immunoglobulin (HBIG), rabies immunoglobulin, tetanus human immunoglobulin (HTIG) and varicella-zoster immunoglobulin (ZIG). Anti-D(Rh_o) immunoglobulin is used to prevent a rhesus-negative mother from forming antibodies to fetal rhesus-positive cells that may reach the maternal circulation, and so protect any further child from the risks of haemolytic disease. An antilymphocyte immunoglobulin obtained from the blood of horses immunized with human lymphocytes is used to prevent the rejection of organ transplants, and its use may permit a reduction in the dose of other immunosuppressive drugs. Antilymphocyte immunoglobulin is also used in transplant rejection crises.

immunosuppressants Drugs such as azathioprine that suppress the normal immune response are used in transplant surgery to prevent tissue rejection, but as their action includes depression of the immune defence system of the body, their use requires care. The systemically acting corticosteroids such as prednisone also have valuable immunosuppressant and cytotoxic properties. Cyclosporin has a powerful immunosuppressant action with little myelotoxicity, and is also used in the prophylaxis of graft-versus-host disease.

indapamide A thiazide-related drug used in hypertension as it has a slow but progressive anti-hypertensive action. *Dose:* 2.5mg daily, continued for some months, until a maximum response has been obtained. Larger doses may merely evoke an increased diuresis. Combined treatment with beta-blocking agents and other drugs may increase the response, but saluretic diuretics are not recommended as they may cause hypokalaemia.

indigo carmine A blue dye that has been used as a 0.4% solution by injection as a renal function test. Normally the urine is coloured blue in 10 minutes or so.

indomethacin A widely used non-steroidal anti-inflammatory and analgesic agent (NSAID) of value in arthritic and rheumatoid conditions, and in acute gout. *Dose:* 50–200mg daily with food. Suppositories 100mg, are useful at night to reduce morning stiffness. Side-effects are numerous and include gastro-intestinal disturbances, which may be severe and cause bleeding; dizziness and confusion. Hypersensitivity reactions with blood disorders have been reported, and blurred vision with corneal deposits may occur with prolonged treatment. Indomethacin is also used by intravenous injection for the closure of the patent ductus arteriosus in premature babies, but the dose requires careful assessment under specialist supervision.

indoramin An alpha-adrenoceptor blocking agent used in hypertension. It has a selective action on the $alpha_1$-receptors, and lowers the blood pressure by reducing the peripheral resistance. The response may be increased by combined treatment with a thiazide diuretic or a beta-blocking agent. *Dose:* 50mg initially daily, increased, if required, up to 200mg daily. It is also used for the symptomatic relief of benign prostatic hypertrophy in doses of 40–100mg daily, although in elderly patients small doses of 20mg at night may be effective. Side-effects include drowsiness, dizziness and some anticholinergic reactions such as dryness of the mouth.

inosine pranobex A complex containing the purine metabolite inosine. The complex has antiviral properties, and may act more by stimulating the immune system of the body than by a direct action on viral replication. Indicated in herpes simplex virus infections of the skin and mucous membranes. *Dose:* 4g daily for 1–2 weeks. Care is necessary in renal impairment, gout or hyperuricaemia.

inositol nicotinate A vasodilator drug used mainly in peripheral vascular disorders such as Raynaud's disease, and acrocyanosis. *Dose:* 1–4g daily.

insulin The antidiabetic principle of the pancreas, regulating the metabolism of carbohydrates and fats. It is widely used in the treatment of diabetes mellitus by subcutaneous injection in doses adjusted to individual need. Many modified insulin products are available, designed to extend the duration of action and reduce the frequency of injections, and so simulate the effects of the natural hormone more closely. Human insulins, obtained by the modification of pork insulin (emp) or by biosynthesis (crb) are also available, and are used routinely to an increasing extent. A transfer from animal to human insulin requires monitoring, and patients should be warned that the usual early symptoms of hypoglycaemia may be less marked. In diabetic emergency, soluble insulin remains the preparation of choice. See Table 11 on page 188.

interferons Proteins formed in mammalian cells in response to viral invasion. When released from infected cells, they protect non-infected cells by preventing the replication of the virus in those cells. Interferons, however, are species-specific, so only human interferon can be used therapeutically. Alpha-interferon has some anti-tumour properties, and is now produced in quantity from cultures of human lymphoblastoid cells, or from *E.coli* cells by recombinant DNA technology. At present, interferon is used mainly in the treatment of hairy-cell leukaemia and AIDS-related Kaposi's sarcoma, but it is also effective against virus papilloma, and may prove to be of value in multiple myeloma and other malignant conditions. It is given by deep intramuscular injection, but the dose varies according to the interferon product used. Side-effects include influenza-like symptoms, anorexia and confusion. Care is necessary in hepatic, renal, cardiovascular or CNS dysfunction.

iodine Powerful antiseptic used as iodine solution, or as povidone-iodine for skin preparation. Hypersensitivity to iodine skin applications are not unknown. Given orally as Lugol's Solution in preoperative treatment of thyrotoxicosis. *Dose:* as Aqueous Iodine Solution (Lugol's solution) 0.1–1ml; as Weak Iodine Solution (tincture of iodine) 0.6–2ml.

iodized oil Poppy-seed oil containing 40% iodine in combination. Used as a contrast agent in lymphangiography, hysterosalpingography, and other radiological examinations.

iodoform Yellow powder with strong odour. Mild antiseptic used occasionally as BIPP.

iopanoic acid A radio-opaque substance used as a contrast agent in cholecystography. It is largely excreted in the bile when given orally. *Dose:* 2–6g.

iophendylate An oily liquid containing 30% of combined iodine. It is mainly used as a contrast agent in myelography. *Dose:* 6–9ml by injection into the subarachnoid space. Before intrauterine blood transfusion, 9ml have been injected into the amniotic sac to outline the fetus. Shock and violent coughing may occur if any iophendylate reaches the circulation.

ipecacuanha The dried root from which emetine is obtained. It has emetic properties, and is used mainly as Ipecacuanha Emetic Mixture. *Dose:* 30ml in adults; 10–15ml in children.

ipratropium An anticholinergic agent with bronchodilator properties. Of value in bronchospasm not responding to selective $beta_2$-receptor stimulants represented by salbutamol. It is relatively free from the side-effects associated with anticholinergic drugs. *Dose:* by aerosol inhalation, 20–40μg (1–2 puffs) four times a day. Similar doses are given by nasal spray in watery rhinorrhoea.

iprindole One of the less sedative tricyclic antidepressants, with the actions and uses of amitriptyline, with reduced anticholinergic and vascular side-effects. *Dose:* 45–90mg daily, increased, if necessary, up to 160mg daily.

iron-dextran, iron-sorbitol Injectable iron products for use when oral iron therapy is not possible or not effective. They are given by deep intramuscular injection in doses based on the degree of iron deficiency. Iron-dextran (but not iron-sorbitol) may be given with care as a single intravenous dose over 6–8 hrs, but such single dose treatment is not without danger.

iron salts See ferrous sulphate.

isoaminile citrate A cough

suppressant used mainly for dry and painful cough. May sometimes cause constipation and nausea. *Dose:* 120–240mg daily as linctus.

isocarboxazid A monoamine oxidase inhibitor with the antidepressant action, uses and side-effects of phenelzine. *Dose:* 30mg initially daily, subsequently increased if necessary up to 60mg daily, reduced later to 10–20mg daily according to need.

isoconazole An antifungal agent similar to miconazole. Used for the single-dose local treatment of candidal and trichomonal vaginal infections. *Dose:* 600mg as 2 vaginal pessaries.

isofluorane An inhalation anaesthetic with the action and uses of halothane and enflurane. It is given as a 0.5–3% oxygen-nitrous oxide mixture from a calibrated vaporizer.

isoniazid A pyridine derivative with a specific action against *Mycobacterium tuberculosis*. Widely used in the treatment of tuberculosis, but as bacterial resistance soon develops, combined treatment with other drugs such as rifampicin is essential. *Dose:* 300mg daily, or 1g twice a week, and often continued for some months. Side-effects include nausea and peripheral neuritis, rash and psychotic episodes.

isoprenaline An orally active adrenaline-related drug with increased bronchodilator and reduced vasoconstrictor potency. It is used in the control of asthma, bronchitis and related conditions. *Dose:* 20–60mg daily as sublingual tablets, or 80–240μg (1–3 puffs) by aerosol inhalation up to eight times a day. It is also given in severe bradycardia and heart block. *Dose:* 90mg or more, up to 840mg daily; dose by intravenous infusion, 1–10μg/minute, as required. Side-effects include nausea, tachycardia, and tremor. Care is necessary in ischaemic heart disease and diabetes.

isosorbide dinitrate A vasodilator with the actions, uses and side-effects of glyceryl trinitrate, but with a more prolonged action. *Dose:* in acute angina, 5–10mg, sublingually; for extended treatment 120mg orally daily; in left ventricular failure up to 240mg daily; by intravenous infusion, 2–10mg/hr.

isosorbide mononitrate The active metabolite of the dinitrate. It escapes first-pass loss in the liver, and has a more rapid action. May cause peripheral vasodilatation and headache. *Dose:* 40–120mg daily.

isotretinoin A potent, orally active derivative of vitamin A. It is used for *severe* acne not responding to other treatment, and brings about a prolonged remission of symptoms. *Dose:* 500μg/kg daily for 4 weeks to assess response, followed by treatment for 8–10 weeks. An exacerbation of symptoms is common after 2–8 weeks, which usually subsides later. Side-effects include dryness of mucous membranes, conjunctivitis, nausea and muscle pain. Isotretinoin is teratogenic, and its use requires care under expert supervision.

isoxsuprine A sympathomimetic agent with a relaxant action on uterine muscle. It is given to delay uncomplicated premature labour by intravenous infusion in doses of 200–300μg/minute initially, increased up to 500μg/minute. To maintain control further doses of 10mg are given by intramuscular injection at intervals of 3–6 hours. Side-effects are nausea, flushing, palpitations and hypotension.

ispaghula The husk of ispaghula seed. It swells in water and is used as a bulk laxative. It is also useful in irritable bowel syndrome and diverticulitis. *Dose:* 3–5g daily.

isradipine A calcium channel blocking agent used in hypertension. *Dose:* 5mg daily initially, increased after 3–4 weeks to 10mg daily, with subsequent adjustment to maintenance doses of 2.5–5mg daily according to response. Side-effects include dizziness, headache, palpitations and local oedema.

itraconazole An orally active antifungal agent used in the treatment of vulvcvaginal candidiasis, pityriasis and tinea infections. *Dose:* 200mg twice a day for the 1-day treatment of vulvovaginal infections; 200mg daily for 7 days in pityriasis, 100mg daily for 15–30 days in tinea infections. Side-effects are nausea and abdominal pain. It is metabolized in the liver, so liver disease is a contraindication.

ivermectin A fungal derivative effective against the microfilaria causing 'river blindness'. It does not kill either the adult worms or their larvae, but prevents the growth of the latter, and treatment must be continued until the adult worms die out. *Dose:* 150μg/kg as a single dose, repeated annually.

K

kanamycin An aminoglycoside antibiotic with the actions, uses and side-effects of that group of drugs. Now used mainly in gentamicin-resistant infections. *Dose:* 1g daily by intramuscular injection; 15–30mg/kg daily by intravenous infusion.

kaolin Aluminium silicate. Used as an adsorbent in diarrhoea, colitis, food poisoning, etc. often as Kaolin and Morphine Mixture. *Dose:* 10–20ml as required. It is also used externally as Kaolin Poultice to relieve the pain of sprains, etc.

Kelocyanor A specific antidote for cyanide poisoning. Contains dicobalt edetate, which when given intravenously binds and inactivates any cyanide in the blood. *Dose:* 300mg by slow intravenous injection.

ketamine A short-acting intravenous anaesthetic with analgesic properties. *Dose:* 1–2mg/kg intraveneously over 1 minute, repeated as required; 4–10mg/kg by deep intramuscular injection. It is used mainly in paediatric anaesthesia, and its analgesic action is also of value in neurodiagnostic procedures, and other painful investigations. Hallucinations may occur during the recovery period.

ketazolam A longer-acting benzodiazepine with the action and side-effects of diazepam. It is used mainly in the short-term treatment of severe anxiety. *Dose:* 15–60mg at night.

ketoconazole A broad-spectrum, orally active antifungal agent. It is of value in systemic and deep mycoses, and in severe and resistant mycoses of the gastrointestinal tract and the vagina. It is also effective in severe mycoses of the skin, but it should be used only for superficial fungal infections not responding to other treatment. *Dose:* 200mg daily with food, up to a maximum of 400mg daily. Side-effects include nausea, rash and pruritus. The use of the drug has been associated with a fatal hepatitis.

ketoprofen A non-steroidal anti-inflammatory and analgesic agent of the ibuprofen type. It is of value in rheumatoid arthritis, gout, spondylitis and related conditions, and in dysmenorrhoea. *Dose:* 100–200mg daily with food; 100mg by suppository at night. Care is necessary in peptic ulcer and hepatic disease. May increase the action of anticoagulants and other drugs bound to plasma protein.

ketorolac A potent analgesic that although related to the NSAIDs, has no anti-inflammatory action. It is used for post-operative pain in doses of 30mg by intramuscular injection, with subsequent doses of 10–30mg 4–6 hrly as required, up to a total of 120mg daily for 5 days. Side-effects are those of NSAIDs. Contra-indicated in peptic ulcer and sensitivity to aspirin and related drugs.

ketotifen An antihistamine that also has some of the properties of sodium cromoglycate. It is used in the prophylactic treatment of asthma. *Dose:* 4mg daily with food, continued for some weeks to obtain maximum response. Other anti-asthmatic therapy should be continued for at least 2 weeks to ensure maintenance of control. Side-effects include sedation and dryness of the mouth.

L

labetalol A beta-adrenoceptor blocking agent with some alpha-blocking activity. Like related drugs, labetalol is indicated in all types of hypertension, including that following myocardial infarction. *Dose:* 400mg daily initially, with food, slowly increased up to a maximum of 2.4g daily; by intravenous injection 50mg; for the rapid control of the hypertension of pregnancy 20–160mg by i.v. infusion hourly. It should be used with care in asthma and heart block. Side-effects include weakness, nausea and rash.

lachesine An atropine-like drug with cycloplegic and mydriatic properties. It is used as eye-drops (1%) in patients hypersensitive to related drugs.

lactic acid The acid present in sour milk. Used mainly as Compound Sodium Lactate Injection (Hartmann's Solution) in acidosis and electrolyte disturbances. The injection solution is sometimes given orally in infantile gastro-enteritis. Calcium lactate is sometimes used in supplementary calcium therapy.

lactoflavin See riboflavine.

lactulose A semi-synthetic sugar that is not absorbed by the gastrointestinal tract, and by increasing faecal bulk it is useful in chronic constipation. It also reduces the activity of colonic ammonia-producing organisms, and so is of value in hepatic encephalopathy. *Dose:* as elixir (3.35g/ml) 30–150ml daily.

laevulose (fructose) An easily digested sugar, particularly for diabetics as it can be converted to glycogen in the absence of insulin. Sometimes given intravenously as an alternative to glucose.

lamotrigine An anti-epileptic that alleviates the imbalance of neurotransmitters in the brain by inhibiting the influx of sodium ions. It is used as additional treatment in seizures not fully controlled by other drugs. *Dose:* 50mg twice daily initially; 200–400mg daily for maintenance.

Half doses should be given with sodium valproate. Side-effects are macropapular rash, and dizziness and drowsiness as with other anti-epileptics. See page 192.

lanatoside C A cardiac glycoside from *Digitalis lanata* which is largely converted into digoxin in the body. *Dose:* 1.5–2mg daily for 3–5 days for digitalization, maintenance dose, 250μg–1mg daily. It is excreted more rapidly than some digitalis products and so has a wider margin of safety.

lanolin Wool fat.

Lassar's paste A stiff ointment containing zinc oxide, starch and white soft paraffin with 2% salicylic acid. Used as protective in eczema.

leucovorin See folinic acid.

leuprorelin A synthetic hormone that indirectly suppresses the testicular formation of androgens by inhibiting gonadotrophin production. It is used in advanced prostatic carcinoma. *Dose:* 3.75mg by subcutaneous or intramuscular injection every 4 weeks, and during remission. Side-effects are impotence, flushing and local irritation and the injection site should be varied. There may be an initial temporary increase in androgen production.

levamisole A well-tolerated, single dose anthelmintic of value in round worm (*Ascaris*). *Dose:* 150mg. It is also effective against hookworm (*Ancylostoma* and *Necator*). *Dose:* 2.5–5mg/kg daily for 2–5 days.

levobunolol A beta-blocker used as eye-drops 0.5% in glaucoma.

levodopa An amino acid that is converted to dopamine in the body. It is used in the treatment of Parkinson's disease, which is associated with a reduction in brain dopamine levels due to degeneration in the substantia nigra, thus causing an imbalance in the neurohormonal system of the brain. Levodopa is essentially replacement therapy, but as an oral dose is metabolized to some extent in the peripheral circulation, it is often given with an enzyme inhibitor such as benserazide or carbidopa. Combined therapy permits a larger dose of active drug to reach the cerebral tissues, and at the same time reduces some of the general side-effects of levodopa. *Dose:* 125–500mg initially, increased according to need and response. Side-effects include nausea and cardiovascular disturbances, but psychiatric side-effects may be dose-limiting. Closed-angle glaucoma is a contra-indication. See page 210.

†**levorphanol** A powerful, morphine-like analgesic with

a reduced sedative activity. It is used in the relief of severe pain, especially in the daytime, when the reduced sedative action may be an advantage. *Dose:* 3–9mg daily; 2–4mg by subcutaneous or intramuscular injection, repeated as required; 1–2mg intravenously. Side-effects are nausea, constipation and confusion. Lower doses are indicated in the elderly.

lignocaine A widely used local anaesthetic. It is used for infiltration anaesthesia as a 0.25–0.5% solution, usually with adrenaline, as well as for epidural, caudal and nerve blocks. It is the local anaesthetic present in many dental cartridges. A 2–4% solution is used for surface anaesthesia, and a 2% gel is used to relieve the pain and discomfort of catheterization. Lignocaine is also the drug of choice in the control of ventricular tachycardia following myocardial infarction. *Dose:* 100mg as an intravenous bolus, followed by a dose of 4 mg/min by intravenous infusion for 30 min, with subsequent doses of 2mg/min. Side-effects include confusion, convulsions, bradycardia and hypotension.

Elma cream contains lignocaine and prilocaine. It is used for intradermal anaesthesia to relieve the pain associated with injections, especially in children. It is applied under an occlusive dressing 1–2 hrs before the injection.

lincomycin An antibiotic with the actions, uses and potential dangers of clindamycin. *Dose:* 2g daily.

lindane A pesticide used as a 1% solution for the treatment of pediculosis and scabies.

liothyronine A thyroid hormone with a rapid action, and probably a precursor of thyroxine. It is given orally in severe hypothyroid conditions when a rapid action is necessary, and by injection in hypothyroid coma. *Dose:* 5–60μg daily; 5–20μg intravenously.

liquid paraffin A lubricant laxative and faecal softener. *Dose:* 10–30ml. The extended use of liquid paraffin is discouraged, as it may cause granulomatous reactions, lipid pneumonia, and reduce the absorption of fat-soluble vitamins.

lisinopril An ACE inhibitor similar to enalapril, but with a longer action that permits the use of a single daily dose. In the treatment of hypertension it is given in doses of 2.5mg daily initially, slowly increased according to response up to 10–20mg daily, occasionally up to 40mg. In patients receiving diuretics, such therapy should be withdrawn for 2–3 days before lisinopril therapy. See page 199.

lithium carbonate Lithium carbonate and citrate are used for their mood-regulating action in the prophylaxis and treatment of mania and depressive illness, but the mode of action is not known. The therapeutic/toxic range of lithium is very narrow, and continuous control of the plasma/lithium level is essential to avoid the many side-effects and hazards of therapy. *Dose:* 0.25–2g daily initially, then adjusted to maintain a lithium/plasma level of 0.6–1.2mmol/litre. Prolonged treatment may be required with an adequate fluid intake. Thiazide diuretics should be avoided. Some slow-release tablets are available, but different products *must not* be regarded as interchangeable. Lithium treatment cards giving advice can be obtained from a pharmacy.

lithium succinate Lithium succinate appears to have some antifungal and anti-inflammatory properties, and is used as an 8% ointment for seborrhoeic dermatitis associated with the yeast *Pityrosporum ovale*.

lofepramine An antidepressant of the imipramine group, with similar actions and uses, but reduced sedative and anticholinergic side-effects. *Dose:* 140–210mg daily.

Lomotil A preparation of diphenoxylate, with atropine, for the rapid control of diarrhoea. *Dose:* 2 tablets 6-hrly.

lomustine A slow-acting cytotoxic agent used in Hodgkin's disease and solid tumours. *Dose:* 130mg/m^2 body surface at intervals of 4–6 weeks. Side-effects include anorexia, nausea, liver damage and myelodepression. Dosage should not be repeated until white cell and platelet counts have returned to an acceptable level. Reduced doses are given when lomustine forms part of a multi-drug dosage scheme.

loperamide A synthetic inhibitor of peristalsis used in the treatment of diarrhoea. *Dose:* in acute diarrhoea, 4mg initially, followed by 2mg as required, up to a maximum of 16mg daily. In chronic diarrhoea, 4–8mg daily, but care is necessary in the elderly to avoid faecal impaction. Loperamide is not suitable for children under 4 years of age, nor in patients with liver disease, as it may cause undesirable sedation.

loprazolam A benzodiazepine hypnotic, used mainly in the short-term treatment of insomnia and nocturnal arousal. *Dose:* 1–2mg at bedtime. Side-effects include drowsiness, dizziness, dry mouth and headache. Care is necessary in glaucoma, respiratory disease, and in renal or hepatic impairment. See page 202.

loratadine An antihistamine with the general action of that group of drugs, but with reduced sedative side-effects. *Dose:* 10mg daily. See page 172.

lorazepam A short-acting anxiolytic/hypnotic similar to diazepam, but less likely to cause next-day drowsiness. *Dose:* 1–4mg daily. It is also given by slow intravenous injection in the control of acute panic attacks in doses of 25–30μg/kg, repeated after 6 hours if necessary.

lormetazepam A short-acting benzodiazepine hypnotic. It is useful in the treatment of insomnia in the elderly, but is less suitable for insomnia associated with early awakening. *Dose:* 500μg–1mg at night.

loxapine Antipsychotic agent with the actions and uses of chlorpromazine. Dose in acute and chronic psychoses 25–50mg daily, slowly increased as required. Maintenance doses range from 20–100mg daily. Side-effects are those of other antipsychotic agents, but loxapine may cause nausea, vomiting and weight changes.

Lugol's solution An aqueous solution of iodine 5% and potassium iodide 10%. Used in the pre-operative treatment of thyrotoxicosis. *Dose:* 0.3–1ml.

lymecycline A soluble complex of tetracycline and lysine. It has the action and uses and side-effects of tetracycline, but is absorbed more readily. *Dose:* 800mg daily.

lynoestrenol A progestogen similar to norethisterone, and a constituent of some oral contraceptive products. See page 278.

lypressin An analogue of vasopressin used to control the polyuria of pituitary diabetes insipidus. *Dose:* 2.5–10 units several times a day by nasal spray. Side-effects include nausea and abdominal pain. Lypressin has some vasoconstrictor properties, and desmopressin is often preferred.

lysuride A new drug for the treatment of parkinsonism, that appears to act like bromocriptine by stimulating surviving dopamine receptors in the brain. *Dose:* 200μg at night with food, increased at weekly intervals according to response up to a maximum of 5mg daily. Side-effects include nausea, dizziness and initial hypotensive reactions. See page 210.

M

macrolides A group of antibiotics that differ chemically from the penicillins, yet have a similar pattern of activity. They are active orally and are useful in the treatment of penicillin-sensitive patients. Erythromycin is the most widely used member of the group, with clarithromycin and azithromycin as recent introductions.

magnesium carbonate A white, insoluble powder with antacid and laxative properties. *Dose:* 0.6–4g daily.

magnesium chloride A soluble magnesium salt that is sometimes given by intravenous infusion in the magnesium deficiency that may arise from prolonged diarrhoea and vomiting, or as a consequence of alcoholism. The dose depends on the plasma magnesium levels reported by the laboratory.

magnesium hydroxide A mild antacid laxative, usually given in aqueous suspension as Cream of Magnesia, although tablet forms are also available. Cream of Magnesia is a useful antidote in mineral acid poisoning.

magnesium sulphate (Epsom salts) A powerful saline aperient, producing loose stools by preventing the reabsorption of water. *Dose:* 5–15g before breakfast. Used externally for the treatment of boils and carbuncles as a paste with glycerin.

magnesium trisilicate A white insoluble powder, with mild but prolonged antacid effects. It is widely employed for the treatment of peptic ulcer, often in association with other antacids. *Dose:* 0.3–2g.

malathion An organophosphorus insecticide. Used as a lotion 0.5% for lice and scabies as alternative to lindane or carbaryl.

Mandl's paint A solution of iodine in glycerin. Used occasionally in tonsillitis as an antiseptic throat paint.

mannitol A sugar that is not metabolized, and is used mainly as an osmotic diuretic. *Dose:* (after a test dose of 200mg/kg) 50–200g by slow intravenous infusion over 24 hours. Mannitol has also been used by intravenous infusion as a short-term ocular hypotensive agent in the treatment of glaucoma. It is also useful for increasing urinary elimination in drug overdose. Care is necessary to maintain fluid balance during treatment.

maprotiline A sedative antidepressant with a general action similar to that of the tricyclic drugs represented by amitriptyline. *Dose:* 25–150mg daily. If given at night as a single dose, the sedative action may reduce the need for other drugs. It has milder anticholinergic side-effects than some related compounds, although skin rash is more common.

†**mazindol** A centrally-acting appetite depressant used in

the short-term treatment of obesity. *Dose:* 2mg daily after breakfast. Side-effects are insomnia, dizziness and dependence.

mebendazole An anthelmintic effective against most intestinal worms. *Dose:* 100mg once for threadworm, and 100mg twice daily for 2 days against other infestations. Generally well tolerated, but it should not be given to children under 2 years of age.

mebeverine An antispasmodic agent which, unlike the anticholinergic drugs, appears to have a direct action on the intestinal smooth muscle. It is useful in the treatment of gastrointestinal spasm and in the irritable bowel syndrome. *Dose:* 400mg daily, before food. As with other antispasmodics, mebeverine should not be used in paralytic ileus.

mebhydrolin An antihistamine used for the symptomatic relief of hayfever, urticaria and other allergic conditions. *Dose:* 150–300mg daily. The side-effects are those of the antihistamines generally.

mecillinam A penicillin that is exceptional in being active against many Gram-negative bacilli, including *E.coli, Proteus, Salmonella* and similar organisms, although *Pseudomonas aeruginosa* remains resistant. It is used mainly in severe Gram-negative infections. *Dose:* 5–15mg/kg by intramuscular or slow intravenous injection 6–8-hrly. Care is necessary in renal dysfunction. See pivmecillinam.

medazepam An anxiolytic benzodiazepine with the action and side-effects of diazepam. *Dose:* 15–30mg daily, increased up to 40mg daily in severe anxiety.

medroxyprogesterone A progestogen used in amenorrhoea and functional uterine bleeding. *Dose:* 2.5–10mg daily. For the control of endometriosis, 50mg weekly by i.m. injection for 6 months or more. In breast cancer and other hormone-dependent neoplasms, much larger doses, both orally and by injection, may be required. For short-term contraception, 150mg once by deep i.m. injection. Care is necessary in patients who have experienced endogenous depression and a recurrence is an indication that the drug should be withdrawn.

mefenamic acid A non-steroidal anti-inflammatory analgesic agent used to relieve moderate pain in arthritic and rheumatoid conditions, and other states requiring mild analgesic therapy such as menorrhagia. *Dose:* 1.5g daily after food. Side-effects are drowsiness, bronchospasm and haemolytic anaemia. Diarrhoea is an indication that the drug should be withdrawn.

mefloquine A new drug for the prophylaxis and treatment of chloroquine-resistant malaria. *Dose:* for short-term prophylaxis 250mg weekly for 6 weeks, starting 1 week before exposure. Doses for treatment require specialist advice. Side-effects include gastro-intestinal disturbances, dizziness and weakness. It is not suitable for use in severe renal or hepatic impairment.

mefruside A diuretic with a slower and more prolonged action than related drugs such as frusemide. Useful in the long-term treatment of oedema, hypertension and pre-menstrual tension. *Dose:* 12.5–50mg daily preferably in the morning, according to need and response. A potassium supplement may be required. Care is necessary in renal and hepatic deficiency.

megestrol An orally active progestogen. It is used in oestrogen-dependent breast cancers, and acts by suppressing the uptake of oestrogens by the cancer cells. *Dose:* 160mg daily. Nausea and fluid retention with weight gain are occasional side-effects.

melphalan A cytotoxic drug with an action similar to mustine. It is used in the treatment of multiple myeloma, ovarian adenocarcinoma, malignant melanoma and other cancerous states. *Dose:* 150–300μg/kg daily for 4–6 days, repeated after 1–2 months. In myeloma it is also given by regional perfusion. The injection solution is highly irritant and contact should be avoided. Side-effects include myelodepression, nausea, rash and pruritus.

menadiol A water-soluble form of vitamin K. Phytomenadione is now preferred.

menotrophin Human menopausal gonadotrophin containing follicle-stimulating hormone and luteinizing hormone. It is used in conjunction with chorionic gonadotrophin in the treatment of anovulatory sterility. The dose depends on individual hormone assays and response. The use of the drug has resulted in multiple births. It is also given to males to stimulate spermatogenesis.

menthol Colourless crystals obtained from oil of peppermint. Used as spray or drops for nasopharyngeal inflammation, and as an inhalation, often with friar's balsam, for the relief of coryza and catarrh.

mepacrine A synthetic antimalarial. Now replaced by chloroquine and other powerful drugs. It is used occasionally in the treatment for *Giardia lamblia* infections. *Dose:* 300mg daily for 5–8 days.

mepenzolate An anticholinergic agent used in the control of gastrointestinal disturbances associated with smooth muscle spasm. *Dose:* 75–200mg daily. Side-effects include dryness of the mouth, blurred vision and bradycardia.

†**meprobamate** A mild tranquillizer used in anxiety and tension states, and in alcoholism, but its extended use may lead to dependence. *Dose:* 1.2–2.4g daily. Side-effects are drowsiness, headache, gastrointestinal and visual disturbances. Care is necessary in epilepsy, as the drug may precipitate seizures. It has been largely replaced by benzodiazepine anxiolytics.

meptazinol An analgesic with a more rapid and extended action than morphine, and less likely to cause respiratory depression. It also has a reduced dependence potential. It is used in moderate to severe pain. *Dose:* 800–1600mg orally daily. In severe pain, 75–100mg by injection, repeated as required; in obstetric analgesia, 2mg/kg. The action can be partly antagonized by naloxone. Side-effects include dizziness and nausea.

mequitazine An antihistamine used for the symptomatic relief of allergic states such as hayfever and urticaria. It is less likely to cause sedation than some other antihistamines. *Dose:* 10mg daily. Side-effects may include dry mouth and blurred vision.

mercaptopurine A cytotoxic agent used in the treatment of acute leukaemia and chronic myelogenous leukaemia. *Dose:* 2.5mg/kg daily. Close haematological control is essential, as the drug has a marked myelosuppressive action. Mercaptopurine is also hepatotoxic, and should be withdrawn if jaundice occurs.

mercuric oxide Mercuric oxide ointment 1% has long been used in superficial eye infections. Its use has declined as more effective drugs have been available.

mesalazine The active metabolite of sulphasalazine, which is used in ulcerative colitis. It is not suitable for oral use as such, but can be given as a resin-drug complex, so that the drug reaches and is released in the colon unchanged. It is used mainly for the maintenance of remission of ulcerative colitis, particularly in patients unable to tolerate sulphasalazine. *Dose:* 1.2–2.4g daily. Side-effects include gastrointestinal disturbances, and care is necessary in patients hypersensitive to salicylates. Lactulose should not be used as a laxative, as it may hinder the release of the active drug.

mesna A compound used to prevent the haemorrhagic cystitis caused by the cytotoxic drugs cyclophosphamide and ifosfamide. The reaction is caused by the metabolite acrolein, and mesna reduces the toxicity by combining with acrolein in the urinary tract. *Dose:* 20% of that of the cytotoxic drug, and should be given at the same time by intravenous injection. Subsequent supportive doses may be given orally or by injection 4–8 hrs after therapy.

mesterolone An orally active androgen with the actions and uses of testosterone. It is used in androgen deficiency and male infertility, but unlike other androgens, it does not inhibit endogenous androgen production, and is less hepatotoxic. *Dose:* 75–100mg daily for some months.

mestranol An orally active oestrogen present in some oral contraceptive products. See page 278.

metaraminol A sympathomimetic agent that increases the blood pressure by a general constriction of the peripheral blood vessels. It is used mainly in the acute hypotension that may occur with spinal anaesthesia. It has also been used in shock, but the use of vasoconstrictors has declined, as in shock the peripheral resistance may be already high, and the use of blood volume expanders and dopamine is now preferred. *Dose:* 2–10mg by intramuscular or subcutaneous injection; 5–100mg by intravenous infusion. Side-effects are tachycardia and reduced renal blood flow. It is contra-indicated in myocardial infarction.

metformin An orally active biguanide hypoglycaemic agent. *Dose:* 1.5g daily, adjusted according to need and response. Its action differs from that of the sulphonylureas, as it acts by increasing the peripheral uptake of glucose. It is used mainly in non-insulin-dependent diabetes not controlled by diet and sulphonylurea therapy. *Dose:* 1.5–3g daily. Side-effects include nausea, and transient diarrhoea. It may cause lactic acidosis in some patients, mainly when some renal failure is present, and the drug should then be withdrawn.

†**methadone** A morphine-like analgesic with reduced sedative effects. Of value in severe pain, and in the relief of useless cough in terminal disease. *Dose:* 5–10mg orally or by intramuscular or subcutaneous injection, at intervals according to need. Prolonged treatment carries the risk of cumulative effects and overdose.

methenamine See hexamine.

methicillin A penicillin active against penicillinase-producing staphylococci, but less active against other organisms. Its use has declined as other and orally active penicillins such as flucloxacillin have become available. *Dose:* 1g i.m. 4–6-hrly.

methionine A sulphur-containing amino acid essential for nutrition. It has been used in toxic hepatitis and to increase the effects of some urinary antiseptics by acidifying the urine. *Dose:* 3–10g daily. Also used in paracetamol poisoning (as an alternative to acetylcysteine). *Dose:* 2.5g 4-hrly up to a total of 10g.

methixene An anticholinergic drug used in the treatment of parkinsonism, although it tends to relieve the tremor more than the rigidity of the disease. *Dose:* 15–60mg daily, reduced if necessary to half doses in elderly patients. The side-effects are similar to those of other anticholinergic drugs. See page 210.

methocarbamol A skeletal muscle relaxant used in fibrositis and muscle injury. *Dose:* 6g daily orally; 1–3g daily by slow intravenous injection. It may cause drowsiness, dizziness and allergic rash. Contra-indicated in glaucoma, epilepsy and prostatic hypertrophy.

methohexitone A short-acting intravenous anaesthetic similar to thiopentone. Although less irritant to the tissues, the induction of anaesthesia may be less smooth. It is used mainly for the induction and maintenance of anaesthesia for short operative procedures, when the quick recovery may be an advantage.

methotrexate A cytotoxic agent that acts by inhibiting the enzyme system controlling the synthesis of purines, and so indirectly interferes with cell proliferation. It is used chiefly for maintenance therapy in the remission of acute lymphoblastic leukaemia in children, but it has been used in choriocarcinoma as well as some lymphomas and solid tumours. *Dose:* in children, 15mg/m^2 weekly. It is sometimes effective in resistant psoriasis, and is given in oral doses of 10–25mg weekly under specialist supervision. Side-effects are those of gastrointestinal toxicity, myelodepression, rash and cirrhosis. Blood counts and liver function tests during treatment are essential. Folinic acid is used in methotrexate toxicity.

methotrimeprazine An anti-psychotic agent of the chlorpromazine type, with similar actions, uses and side-effects. It is used in schizophrenia when a sedative effect is also required. *Dose:* 25–50mg daily, but much larger doses, up to 1g daily, may be required, particularly for bedfast patients. It is of value as an adjunct to other therapy in terminal illness and is sometimes given by continuous subcutaneous infusion in doses of 25–200mg over 24 hrs.

methoxamine A sympathomimetic agent that increases the blood pressure by constriction of the peripheral vessels. It is used in the hypotension following spinal anaesthesia; to correct an excessive response to antihypertensive drugs, and to arrest supraventricular tachycardia. *Dose:* 5–20mg by intramuscular injection; 5–10mg by slow intravenous injection. Care is necessary in pre-existing hypertension and cardio-vascular disease.

methyclothiazide A diuretic with the actions, uses and side-effects of bendrofluazide. *Dose:* 2.5–10mg as a single morning dose.

methyl cellulose A derivative of cellulose that is used as an emulsifying agent and bulk laxative. *Dose:* 1.5–6g with water, but not at night. It is sometimes given in diarrhoea, with a minimum amount of water.

methyl salicylate A pale yellow liquid with a characteristic odour. It has long been used as liniment and ointment for the local relief of muscle pain and rheumatic conditions.

methylated spirit Alcohol containing 5% of wood naphtha. Used for skin preparation and alcoholic applications. The methylated spirit used domestically differs, and is coloured violet to indicate its unsuitability for medicinal use.

methylcysteine A sputum-liquefier claimed to be of value in respiratory conditions where the sputum is viscid. *Dose:* 600mg daily.

methyldopa A centrally acting antihypertensive drug, usually given together with a diuretic. It has the advantage of being relatively safe in asthma, heart failure and pregnancy. *Dose:* 1.5–3g daily; 250–500mg by intravenous infusion. Side-effects are drowsiness, depression and diarrhoea. A systemic lupus erythematosus-like syndrome may also occur, and active liver disease is a contra-indication.

†**methylphenobarbitone** An anticonvulsant with the actions, uses and side-effects of phenobarbitone. Dose in epilepsy: 100–600mg daily.

methylprednisolone A corticosteroid with the actions, uses and side-effects of prednisolone, and given in similar doses.

methysergide A synthetic drug

related to ergometrine and used in the prevention of severe and recurrent migraine not responding to other drugs. *Dose:* 2–6mg daily. It is also given for the control of the carcinoid syndrome in doses of 12–20mg daily. Methysergide has many side-effects, including retroperitoneal and cardiac fibrosis, and its use require expert supervision. See page 204.

metipranolol A beta-adrenoceptor blocking agent used as eye-drops 0.1–0.6% for the treatment of chronic glaucoma.

metirosine An enzyme inhibitor that interferes with the synthesis of adrenaline and other pressor amines. It is used mainly in the pre-operative control of adrenaline-producing tumours (phaeochromocytoma), and in the long-term treatment of patients unsuitable for surgery. *Dose:* 1g daily initially, increased if necessary up to 4g daily. An adequate fluid intake is essential. Side-effects include sedation, which may be marked initially, diarrhoea, which may be severe, depression and confusion.

metoclopramide A stimulant of gastric and small intestine transport. It is used in the treatment of nausea and vomiting generally, including that induced by drugs or migraine, in non-ulcer dyspepsia, and in accelerating the passage of a barium meal. *Dose:* 15–30mg daily; in vomiting due to cytotoxic drugs (preferably before chemotherapy is commenced), 2mg/kg up to a total of 10mg/kg over 24 hrs may be given by intravenous infusion. A single dose of 10–20mg is given by intramuscular or intravenous injection ten minutes before radiological examination. Side-effects include extrapyramidal reactions, facial spasms and oculogyric crises, mainly in young persons, and it is best avoided in patients under 20 years of age. See page 208.

metolazone A diuretic with the actions, uses and side-effects of bendrofluazide. *Dose:* in hypertension, 5mg daily initially; in oedematous states doses up to 80mg daily have been given. It may cause hypokalaemia, requiring supplementary potassium, and cardiac arrhythmias may occur.

metoprolol A beta-blocking agent used in the control of angina, but also of value in hypertension and the prophylaxis of migraine. *Dose:* in angina 100–300mg daily, in hypertension 100–400mg daily, in migraine prophylaxis and thyrotoxicosis 200mg daily. Care is necessary in heart block, bradycardia and pulmonary disease. Occasionally given by slow intravenous injection in acute cardiac arrhythmias. *Dose:* 1–2mg/minute, up to a total of 10–15mg.

metriphonate An organophosphorus schistosomicide, but used only in infections of the hookworm *Schistosoma haemobium*, which is found in the genitourinary veins. *Dose:* orally, in three doses of 7.5mg/kg at intervals of 2–4 weeks.

metronidazole An orally effective drug used in trichomoniasis, amoebiasis and in infections due to anaerobic bacteria. *Dose:* in bacterial and trichomonal vaginitis 600mg daily for 7 days, or as a single dose of 2g. In acute intestinal amoebiasis, 2.4g daily for 5 days. In the prophylaxis and treatment of infections caused by colonic anaerobic pathogens such as *Bacteroides fragilis*, as well as infections by some Gram-negative organisms, metronidazole is given in doses of 1.2g daily orally, or as 1g suppositories. In severe infections, doses of 1.5g are given daily by intravenous infusion, replaced by oral therapy as soon as possible. In *Giardia lamblia* infections, 2g daily for 3 days. Metronidazole is also valuable in pseudomembranous colitis (see clindamycin). Side-effects are mainly gastrointestinal disturbances and can be reduced by giving the dose with food, but epileptiform seizures may occur with high doses, and the drug may cause a disulfiram-type reaction if alcohol is taken.

metyrapone An inhibitor of glucocorticoid synthesis, and is used as a test of adrenal cortex function. When metyrapone is given, the plasma concentration of glucocorticoids falls, which then stimulates the production of corticotrophin by the anterior pituitary gland, which in turn stimulates the adrenal cortex to synthesize and release corticosteroid precursors. A rise in the urinary concentration of such precursors is indicative of an active gland. *Dose:* 750mg 4-hrly for 6 doses. For treatment of resistant oedema due to increased aldosterone production, 2.5–4.5g daily. It is also used in the control of Cushing's syndrome. Nausea and vomiting are side-effects.

mexenone A benzophenone derivative that absorbs ultraviolet light. Used as a 4% cream for protection against sunburn.

mexiletine An anti-arrhythmic drug that is useful in the control of ventricular arrhythmias, particularly those following myocardial infarction, or when lignocaine is ineffective. *Dose:* as a loading dose, 100–250mg intravenously, followed by i.v. infusion of a 0.1% solution until a further 250mg has been given. Oral therapy: a loading dose of 400mg, followed by 600mg–1g daily. Side-effects are nausea, drowsiness, confusion and blurred vision. Contra-indicated in bradycardia, hypotension, and hepatic or renal failure.

mezlocillin An antibiotic with a wide range of activity that includes Gram-negative organisms such as *Pseudomonas*, *Proteus* and *Bacteroides fragilis*. Useful in a wide range of systemic and local infections. *Dose:* in severe infections up to 20g daily by intravenous infusion, in less severe infections, 6–8g daily; 1–2g can be given by deep intramuscular injection. For pre-operative prophylaxis doses of 5g have been given intravenously. Lower doses are necessary in renal insufficiency. Penicillin hypersensitivity is a contra-indication.

mianserin An antidepressant of the amitriptyline type, with reduced anticholinergic and cardiovascular side-effects, and well tolerated by the elderly. It is of value in all types of depression, including those associated with anxiety. *Dose:* 30–90mg daily, which may be taken as a single dose at night, although higher doses have been given. Care is necessary in recent myocardial infarction and heart block. Severe hepatic disease is a contra-indication. Side-effects include aplastic anaemia, and blood counts during treatment are essential. The drug should be withdrawn if any signs of infection occur.

miconazole An antifungal agent of value in systemic and alimentary fungal infections. *Dose:* 1g daily orally, or up to 1.8g daily by intravenous infusion, and the duration of treatment largely depends on the response. Pessaries of 100mg and a cream (2%) are used for vaginal candidiasis. A gel is available for oral fungal infections. Side-effects after systemic use include nausea, pruritus and rash. Miconazole may potentiate the action of anticoagulant, anticonvulsant and hypoglycaemic drugs, requiring an adjustment of dose.

midazolam A sedative of the benzodiazepine group, used mainly for sedation before and during gastroscopy, endoscopy and other investigations. The action is rapid, and an anterograde amnesia often follows. *Dose:* by slow intravenous injection 70μg/kg up to a total of 2.5–7mg. Premedication, 2.5–5mg intramuscularly. For the induction of anaesthesia in poor-risk patients, 100–300μg/kg by slow intravenous injection. Side-effects after intravenous injection include respiratory depression and, occasionally, severe hypotension.

mifepristone An antiprogestational agent used as an alternative to surgery for the termination of pregnancy, up to 63 days gestation. Given as a single oral dose of 600mg. For hospital use only.

milrinone An inhibitor of phosphodiesterase, an enzyme concerned in cardiac function. It has a digoxin-like effect on the myocardium, and may be effective in congestive heart failure not responding to other drugs. It is given by intravenous infusion as an initial dose of 50μg/kg, with maintenance doses of 0.5μg/min up to a total dose of 1.13mg over 24 hrs. Side-effects are anginal pain, hypotension and headache. See enoximone.

minocycline A tetracycline with the general properties of that group of antibiotics, but differing as the absorption of minocycline is little influenced by food. It is also suitable for use when the renal function is impaired, as accumulation of the drug is unlikely. *Dose:* 200mg daily. The side-effects are those of the tetracyclines generally, although minocycline may also cause dizziness, vertigo and rash.

minoxidil A vasodilator used in severe hypertension resistant to other drugs. The vasodilatation is linked with water and salt retention, and tachycardia may occur and combined treatment with a beta-blocker and a diuretic is normally required. *Dose:* 5–50mg daily. Side-effects are weight gain and breast tenderness. Almost all patients experience hypertrichosis, and should be warned accordingly. A 2% solution is used as a lotion in the local treatment of male-pattern baldness.

misoprostol A synthetic prostaglandin with an inhibitory action on gastric secretion. It is used in the control of peptic ulcer, and in the prophylaxis of ulcers induced by NSAIDs. *Dose:* 800mg daily with food, with a last dose at night, and continued for some weeks. Dose in prophylaxis 400–800mg daily. Side-effects are usually transient, and include diarrhoea, nausea and abdominal pain. See page 212.

mithramycin See plicamycin.

mitobronitol A cytotoxic agent with an action similar to that of busulphan and used mainly in chronic myeloid leukaemia. *Dose:* 250mg daily until the white cell count falls, then 125mg daily according to need. May cause gastro-intestinal disturbance, alopecia and bone marrow depression, and haematological control is necessary.

mitozantrone A cytotoxic drug related to doxorubicin, and indicated in advanced breast cancer. *Dose:* 14mg/m^2 once i.v., repeated after 21 days, provided the white cell and platelets counts have returned to normal. It is highly irritant, and contact of the drug with the skin must be avoided. Side-effects are nausea, vomiting, alopecia, myelosuppression and cardiac weakness.

monoamine oxidase inhibitors Monoamine oxidase is an enzyme concerned with the breakdown of dopamine, serotonin, noradrenaline and adrenaline. Chemically, these substances are amines, and they are stored in many organs of the body, including the brain, where they function as transmitters of nerve impulses. The period for which they act is very short, as they are rapidly metabolized by monoamine oxidase. An inhibition of the enzyme could permit an increase in the brain levels of such amines, and on that basis some enzyme inhibitors have been used in the treatment of depression. Therapy is complicated by the fact that these drugs can increase the response to pressor drugs, anaesthetics and many other drugs, including the mild sympathomimetics present in some cough mixtures and decongestive nasal sprays. Even certain foods, particularly cheese, may cause a dangerous rise in blood pressure during monoamine oxidase inhibitor therapy and patients should always carry the monoamine oxidase inhibitor warning card. Great care is necessary during combined therapy, and ideally 10–14 days should elapse after ceasing monoamine oxidase inhibitor treatment before using other potent drugs. Examples of monoamine oxidase inhibitors are isocarboxazid, phenelzine and tranylcypromine. Their use has declined as more effective antidepressants of the amitriptyline type, with fewer side-effects, have become available. See page 185.

monosulfiram A useful parasiticide. In scabies, a 25% solution is diluted two or three times with water, and applied after a bath to the whole body, except face and scalp. Also used as a 5% soap for prophylaxis and control in schools.

†**morphine** The principal alkaloid of opium. It is widely used as a narcotic analgesic for the relief of severe pain and the associated anxiety and stress, and in shock. *Dose:* in acute pain, 10mg by injection as required; in chronic pain it may be given

orally or by injection according to need in doses varying from 5–20mg. Some long-acting oral and injectable forms of morphine are available, designed to reduce the frequency of dosing in conditions of severe pain. Side-effects include nausea and vomiting, which can often be controlled by small doses of chlorpromazine, or a similar anti-emetic. Morphine may cause respiratory depression, and severe respiratory depression is a contra-indication. The possibility of tolerance to and dependence on morphine should be kept in mind if treatment is prolonged, but in terminal conditions this is of reduced importance.

†**MST Continus** A sustained release oral preparation of morphine for the prolonged relief of severe pain. Tablets of 10–100mg are available. *Dose:* 10–20mg initially, increased according to need and response.

mupirocin An antibacterial agent that is effective against most of the pathogens responsible for skin infections. It is used as a 2% ointment in impetigo, folliculitis and similar conditions. It may cause some local irritation.

mustine A cytotoxic drug used mainly in the treatment of Hodgkin's disease and related conditions. *Dose:* 0.1mg/kg daily for three days as a fast-running intravenous infusion, or as a single dose of 0.4mg/kg. The solution, which must be freshly prepared, is highly irritant, and extra-venous injection causes very severe local necrosis. It has also been given by intrapleural injection in the control of malignant effusions. The local application of a solution (20mg/100ml) has been used in mycosis fungoides. Side-effects include severe vomiting, bone marrow depression and alopecia. Close haematological control during treatment is essential.

N

nabilone An anti-emetic used in the treatment of nausea and vomiting associated with cancer chemotherapy. *Dose:* 2–4mg daily, beginning the day before cytotoxic treatment is commenced, and continued for a day after the end of the course. Side-effects are drowsiness, confusion and tremor. Care is necessary in liver dysfunction or any history ot psychotic illness. See page 208.

nabumetone A non-acidic anti-inflammatory agent. It is a pro-drug with a relatively weak action but after absorption it is converted into a more active metabolite. It is effective in rheumatoid and osteoarthritis, and its reduced gastric irritant properties appear to be linked with its pro-drug nature. *Dose:* 1g at night. Reduced doses are necessary in renal impairment, and the dose of any oral anticoagulant or hypoglycaemic agent may require adjustment. Contra-indicated in active peptic ulcer.

nadolol A beta-blocking agent with the actions and uses of propranolol. *Dose:* in angina, 40mg daily, or more; in hypertension, 80mg daily, increased slowly as required; in the prophylaxis and treatment of migraine, 80–160mg daily. Maximum daily dose 240mg.

nafarelin A synthetic suppressant of steroid production by the gonads, and used in the treatment of endometriosis. It is given as a once-only course of treatment by nasal spray in doses of 200μg twice a day, starting between the 2nd and 4th day of the menstrual cycle, and continued for up to 6 months. Side-effects are numerous and of the menopausal type.

naftidrofuryl A peripheral and cerebral vasodilator. Claimed to be of value in cerebrovascular disorders. *Dose:* 300–600mg daily. In peripheral vascular disease with ischaemia and incipient gangrene, doses of 200mg twice a day have been given by very slow intravenous infusion. Atrio-ventricular block is a contra-indication.

nalbuphine An opioid analgesic, comparable with morphine in potency, but with reduced side-effects and a reduced dependence potential. *Dose:* by injection, 10–20mg as required. It may cause nausea and dizziness, and care is necessary in respiratory, renal or hepatic dysfunction.

nalidixic acid A synthetic antibacterial agent used in cystitis and infections of the lower urinary tract, especially those due to Gram-negative bacteria (except *Pseudomonas*). It is not suitable for systemic infections, as the blood levels reached with nalidixic acid are too low to be effective. *Dose:* 4g daily for 7 days, with subsequent doses of 2g daily. Side-effects are nausea, visual disturbance, rash, jaundice and phototoxicity. Exposure to sunlight should be avoided; epilepsy is a contra-indication.

naloxone A powerful and rapidly acting antagonist of opioid narcotics. It is used immediately after operation to reduce any narcotic-induced respiratory depression. *Dose:* 100–200μg intravenously initially, followed by 100μg at 2 minute intervals, as required. For neonates, 10μg/kg by injection are given. In narcotic analgesic overdose, 800μg–2mg may be given, up to a total dose of 10mg.

naltrexone A long-acting narcotic antagonist used only to prevent relapse and maintain recovery from opioid addition. It prevents re-addiction only whilst the drug is being taken. *Dose:* 25mg initially, later up to 50mg daily. It must not be given to patients who are still opioid-dependent as an acute withdrawal syndrome may be precipitated.

nandrolone An anabolic steroid related to testosterone, with markedly reduced virilizing properties. It has the anabolic or tissue-building properties of the parent compound, and is used in post-operative convalescence, osteoporosis and wasting diseases. It is sometimes effective in aplastic anaemia, and has been used in the treatment of metastatic breast cancer. *Dose:* 50mg weekly by deep intramuscular injection.

naproxen A widely used non-steroidal anti-inflammatory agent (NSAID) for the relief of rheumatic and musculoskeletal disorders. *Dose:* 0.5–1g daily, increased up to 2g daily in severe conditions. Suppositories of 500mg are useful at night to reduce morning stiffness. Side-effects include headache, dizziness, and dyspepsia with occasional bleeding. Blurred vision may also occur, as well as hypersensitivity reactions such as rash and bronchospasm. Care is necessary in renal and hepatic impairment; peptic ulcer is a contra-indication.

natamycin An antifungal antibiotic. *Dose:* in respiratory fungal infections, 2.5mg by aerosol inhalation; as a cream 2%, as 25mg vaginal tablets in trichomoniasis.

nedocromil An inhibitor of the release of inflammatory mediators in the respiratory tract. It is used in the prophylactic treatment of asthma, but it is not effective in an established attack. *Dose:* by aerosol inhalation, 8mg (4 puffs) daily. Side-effects are transient nausea and headache.

nefopam A powerful analgesic chemically unrelated to other analgesics. It causes little respiratory depression in standard doses. Useful in acute or chronic pain as an alternative to the morphine-type analgesics. *Dose:* 90–270mg daily; 20mg by intramuscular injection. Side-effects include drowsiness, headache and tachycardia. Care is necessary in hepatic disease.

neomycin An antibiotic with a wide range of activity against Gram-positive and Gram-negative bacteria, but it is too toxic for systemic use. It is used mainly as an ointment or cream (0.5%), often with an anti-inflammatory steroid, in infected skin conditions. It is also used locally for ear and eye infections as drops (0.5%), and it is occasionally given orally in doses of 6g daily before bowel surgery. Extended local use may cause allergic reactions, and occasionally ototoxicity.

neostigmine An inhibitor of cholinesterase which thus indirectly prolongs the action of acetylcholine released at nerve endings. It is used mainly in the treatment of myasthenia gravis. *Dose:* 75–300mg daily; 1–2.5mg daily by injection. Side-effects are nausea, salivation, diarrhoea and abdominal cramp, and supplementary treatment with an anticholinergic drug may be required. It is also used post-operatively to antagonize the residual effects of muscle relaxants of the tubocurarine type. *Dose:* 1–5mg intravenously, after a preliminary injection of 0.5–1mg of atropine. It is contra-indicated in urinary or intestinal obstruction.

netilmicin An aminoglycoside antibiotic, less toxic than related drugs. Used mainly in severe infections of the urinary and respiratory tracts that are resistant to gentamicin. *Dose:* 4–6mg/kg daily by intramuscular or intravenous injection. Side-effects are dizziness, vertigo, malaise and rash; ototoxicity may also occur.

neuromuscular blocking agents Drugs used to induce adequate muscle relaxation under a light plane of anaesthesia to facilitate surgery. The non-depolarizing agents such as tubocurarine compete with acetylcholine at the neuromuscular receptor site, and have a relatively long action that can be reversed by neostigmine. The depolarizing relaxants, such as suxamethonium, have an acetylcholine-like action on the receptor site, but as they are broken down less rapidly than acetylcholine, they delay the return of the ability of the muscle to contract again. The action of suxamethonium cannot be reversed by neostigmine.

niacin See nicotinic acid.

nicardipine A calcium-channel blocking agent with a coronary vasodilator action similar to that of verapamil, but with reduced anti-arrhythmic activity. It is used mainly in angina and hypertension, and may be given to patients already receiving beta-blockers. *Dose:* 60–120mg daily. Aortic stenosis is a contra-indication. Side-effects are dizziness, flushing, nausea and palpitations.

niclosamide A synthetic anthelmintic of value in the

elimination of tapeworm. *Dose:* after fasting 2g followed 2 hours later by a purge. It has a toxic effect on the worm, which is killed by the drug. Pruritus is an occasional side-effect.

nicofuranose A nicotinic acid derivative. It has an extended action of some value in peripheral vascular disorders. It is also used in the treatment of hyperlipidaemia, as it has some effect in lowering plasma cholesterol levels. *Dose:* 1.5–3g daily. Side-effects include flushing and dizziness.

nicotinamide A compound derived from nicotinic acid, possessing similar properties, but differing in that it has little vasodilator action. It is useful in deficiency states as well as in pellagra when the vasodilator action of nicotinic acid limits the dose.

nicotinic acid An essential food factor, occurring in yeast, liver, etc, but now prepared synthetically. It is a specific in the treatment of pellagra. It causes vasodilatation, and has been used in Ménière's disease and chilblains, but with variable results. In large doses it reduces the plasma levels of some lipoproteins. *Dose:* 10–30mg daily for prophylaxis; therapeutic dose in pellagra, 250–500mg daily. In hyperlipidaemia, up to 6g daily have been given. Side-effects include flushing, dizziness and pruritus. See page 197.

nicotinyl alcohol A derivative with the vasodilator properties of nicotinic acid, but they are less intense. Useful in peripheral circulatory disturbances such as Raynaud's disease and acrocyanosis. *Dose:* 100–200mg daily.

nicoumalone A synthetic anticoagulant similar to phenindione, and used mainly in the treatment of deep-vein thrombosis. *Dose:* 8–12mg initially, subsequent doses are based on the response, as shown by determination of the blood prothrombin time, expressed as the International Normalized Ratio (INR). Haemorrhage is a potential side-effect.

nifedipine A calcium-channel blocking agent similar to verapamil, but with a more powerful peripheral and coronary vasodilator action. It is used in the treatment of angina, hypertension and Raynaud's disease, and may be given, if required in association with a beta-blocking agent. *Dose:* in angina, 30–60mg daily; in hypertension 40–80mg daily. Side-effects are flushing and headache, which are usually transient, and some ankle oedema may occur. It should be withdrawn if anginal pain develops.

nikethamide A centrally acting respiratory stimulant with mild vasoconstrictor properties. *Dose:* in acute respiratory failure, 0.5–1g by slow intravenous injection. Care is necessary, as the margin between the therapeutic dose and the toxic dose causing convulsions is narrow. Nikethamide is not indicated in respiratory failure due to drug overdose.

nimodipine A calcium channel blocking agent that acts preferentially on the cerebral vessels. It is used in subarachnoid haemorrhage to prevent ischaemic sequelae. Dose within 4 days of onset: 60mg 4-hrly, continued for 21 days. Dose for treatment: 1mg/hr initially by intravenous infusion, increased later to 2mg/hr for 5 days. Side-effects are flushing, hypotension and gastro-intestinal disturbances.

nimorazole An orally active trichomonicide. *Dose:* in trichomoniasis a single dose of 2g with the main meal; in Vincent's gingivitis 500mg twice a day for 2 days. Side-effects are nausea and drowsiness, and an intolerance to alcohol may develop. Contra-indicated in severe renal disease and in neurological disorders.

nitrazepam A benzodiazepine, used as a mild hypnotic when some degree of daytime sedation is acceptable. *Dose:* 5–10mg at night, with reduced doses for elderly patients, and in renal and hepatic dysfunction. Care is necessary in respiratory depression. Some dependence on nitrazepam may occur with extended treatment. The combined use of alcohol increases the hypnotic action.

Nitrocine A solution of glyceryl trinitrate, for intravenous infusion in myocardial ischaemia and refractory angina.

nitrofurantoin An antibacterial agent with a wide range of activity against the majority of urinary pathogens. It is of value in cystitis and pyelitis, and in renal infections that have become resistant to other drugs. It is also used prophylactically but extended use requires care. *Dose:* 400mg daily; 50–100mg at night for prophylaxis. It is ineffective in an alkaline urine. Nausea, rash and peripheral neuropathy are side-effects, and pulmonary infiltration has been reported.

nitrogen mustard See mustine.

nitroglycerine See glyceryl trinitrate.

nitrous oxide The oldest inhalation anaesthetic. Supplied in blue cylinders, it is widely used for brief operative work, and as a 50% oxygen mixture it is used as an inhalation analgesic in obstetrics.

nizatidine A potent and selective H_2-receptor antagonist chemically distinct from cimetidine or ranitidine. It is used in the treatment of benign duodenal and gastric ulcer in single doses of 300mg daily, taken in the evening, or 150mg twice a day, and continued for 4 weeks, or for 8 weeks in gastric ulcer. For prophylactic maintenance treatment, doses of 150mg daily may be given and continued for 12 months. Reduced doses should be given in renal impairment. Reported side-effects include headache, myalgia, cough, pruritus and abnormal dreams.

non-steroidal anti-inflammatory drugs (NSAIDs) Drugs with an anti-inflammatory-analgesic action. The oldest drug in current use is aspirin, but newer compounds, represented by naproxen, diflunisal and indomethacin, are often preferred. They exert their effects by inhibiting the biosynthesis of prostaglandins. In small doses they have a mild analgesic action, but in larger doses the anti-inflammatory action is useful in rheumatoid and arthritic conditions, sports injuries and other inflammatory states. They may cause gastrointestinal disturbances, and should always be taken with food. Hypersensitivity may occur, as well as dizziness, vertigo and bronchospasm. Blood disorders occur occasionally. A balance between the differences in response and the nature of the side-effects may determine the choice of drug. See page 214.

noradrenaline The pressor hormone released at sympathetic nerve endings when such nerves are stimulated. It is also present with adrenaline in the medulla of the adrenal gland. It raises blood pressure mainly by a general vasoconstriction, whereas adrenaline increases the blood pressure by constricting the peripheral vessels and increasing the cardiac output. Noradrenaline is given by slow intravenous infusion in the treatment of shock, peripheral failure, and low blood pressure states, but the response may fluctuate with small variations in dose. The value of vasoconstrictors in shock is now questioned, as in shock the peripheral resistance may well be high, and the blood supply to essential organs such as the kidneys may be reduced. *Dose:* 2–20μg/min, based on need and response. Great care must be taken to avoid extra-venous injection.

norethisterone An orally active progestogen. Used in amenorrhoea, functional uterine bleeding and dysmenorrhoea.

Dose: 5–20mg daily. In breast cancer, large doses up to 60mg daily have been used. To postpone menstruation, 15mg daily for 3 days have been used. In small doses, and in association with an oestrogen, norethisterone and related drugs are widely used as oral contraceptives. See page 278.

norfloxacin A quinolone antibiotic with the actions, uses and side-effects of cinoxacin and other quinolones. Dose in acute urinary tract infections: 800mg daily for 3–10 days: in chronic infections continued for up to 12 weeks. Also used in eye infections as 0.3% drops.

norgestrel Also referred to as levonorgestrel. An orally active progesterone-like drug, and inhibitor of ovulation. Used as a constituent of mixed oral contraceptive products, and as a 'progestogen-only' oral contraceptive. See page 278.

nortriptyline A tricyclic antidepressant with actions, uses and side-effects similar to those of amitriptyline, but with a reduced sedative activity. *Dose:* 20–100mg daily. It is given in nocturnal enuresis in doses of 10–20mg nightly, but the duration of treatment should not exceed 3 months.

noxythiolin A urea derivative with antibacterial properties. It is used in the treatment of bladder infections by the instillation of 100ml of a 2.5% solution. The instillation may cause a burning sensation, and the addition of a local anaesthetic such as amethocaine, to the solution is usually necessary.

NSAIDs See non-steroidal anti-inflammatory drugs.

nystatin A fungicidal antibiotic, used in the treatment of intestinal, vaginal and superficial candidiasis. Oral tablets contain 500 000 units, pessaries contain 100 000 units; cream and ointment 1%. *Oral dose:* 2 million units daily. It is also used as pastilles of 100 000 units for mouth infections.

O

octreotide A synthetic compound that inhibits the release of the growth hormone. It is used in acromegaly, which is caused by an overproduction of the growth hormone by a pituitary tumour. It is given in doses of 100–200μg 8-hrly by subcutaneous injection. It is also used in the symptomatic treatment of the carcinoid syndrome, in which the release of vasoactive substances by a gastro-pancreatic tumour causes flushing and severe diarrhoea. *Dose:* 50μg by subcutaneous injection, increased as needed up to 600μg daily. It has no action on the cause of the syndrome.

oestradiol The oestrogenic hormone controlling ovulation and menstruation. It is used mainly in the control of menopausal symptoms. *Dose:* 10–20μg daily. For prolonged oestrogen replacement therapy, subcutaneous implants containing 25, 50 or 100mg are available. The duration of action of such implants tend to vary, and further implants may be needed after 4–8 months. Skin patches containing 25–100μg of oestradial are also available for hormone replacement therapy. They are usually applied twice weekly. Side-effects are nausea, weight gain, rash and jaundice.

oestriol A natural oestrogen used to relieve the atrophic vaginitis and kraurosis vulvae associated with the decline in the production of oestrogens in the menopause. *Dose:* 250–500mg daily.

olsalazine A compound formed from mesalazine, and used in the treatment of ulcerative colitis. It is more slowly absorbed, and reaches the colon largely unchanged, where it is broken down by intestinal bacteria to release the active metabolite mesalazine. *Dose:* 1–3g daily in acute mild ulcerative colitis; 1g daily for maintenance, often for long periods. The common side-effect is a watery diarrhoea. Salicylate sensitivity is a contra-indication.

omeprazole An inhibitor of the enzyme H^+K^+ATPase. That enzyme controls the final stage of gastric acid production, and its inhibition by omeprazole is of value in conditions resistant to H_2 receptor antagonists, and in reflux oesophagitis, where such agents are not always effective. Dose in benign gastric and duodenal ulcer 20–40mg as a single daily dose for 4–8 weeks. Larger doses may be required in the Zollinger–Ellison syndrome. Side-effects such as nausea, gastro-intestinal disturbances and headache are usually mild.

†Omnopon A preparation of opium alkaloids similar to papaveretum.

ondansetron A potent anti-emetic, of value in the nausea and vomiting associated with cancer chemotherapy. Such vomiting appears to be induced by the release of serotonin, which acts on receptors in the gut as well as stimulating the chemoreceptor trigger zone in the brain. Ondansetron is a specific serotonin blocking agent, and is given before the commencement of cytotoxic or radiotherapy. *Dose:* 24mg daily; in severe vomiting an initial dose of 8mg is given by slow intravenous injection, followed by 1mg/hr for 24 hrs by continuous intravenous infusion, followed by oral therapy. Side-effects are an initial sense of warmth, headache and constipation. See page 208.

†**opium** The dried juice from the capsules of the opium poppy; a brown powder containing 10% of morphine. The action of opium is mainly that of its principal constituent, morphine, but the other alkaloids present modify the action, and opium is preferred to morphine when a constipating action is required, as in intestinal disorders. *Dose:* 30–200mg.

orciprenaline A sympathomimetic agent with the bronchodilator properties of isoprenaline, but with reduced cardiac side-effects. It is used for the relief of obstructive airway conditions. *Dose:* up to 80mg daily; by aerosol inhalation up to 12 puffs (9mg) daily. Side-effects include tremor and tachycardia.

orphenadrine A spasmolytic drug, used in the treatment of parkinsonism, and for the relief of voluntary muscle spasm associated with injury. *Dose:* 200–400mg daily. It may also be given by intramuscular injection in doses of 20–60mg. In parkinsonism it tends to control the rigidity more than the tremor. Side-effects are anticholinergic and include dryness of the mouth, dizziness, visual disturbances. Weight gain has occurred with high doses.

oxamniquine A schistosomicide of low toxicity, but effective only against *Schistosoma mansoni*, found in the veins of the colon and mesentery. It is given in doses of 15–30mg/kg daily for 2–3 days.

oxatomide An antihistamine said to have mast-cell stabilizing properties. Useful in allergic rhinitis, urticaria and similar conditions. *Dose:* 60–120mg daily. May cause drowsiness.

oxazepam A benzodiazepine with the actions, uses and side-effects of diazepam. It is useful in acute anxiety and panic states. *Dose:* 45–120mg daily.

oxerutins A mixture of rutosides (flavonoid derivatives) which is claimed to reduce capillary fragility and permeability. It has been used in venous disorders of the lower limbs. *Dose:* 750–1000mg daily.

oxitropium An anticholinergic bronchodilator similar to ipratropium, and used by aerosol inhalation in stable chronic asthma and related conditions. *Dose:* 200–300μg

(4–6 puffs) daily.

oxpentifylline An aminophylline-like drug used mainly as a vasodilator in peripheral vascular disorders. *Dose:* 800–1200mg. It may cause nausea, flushing and dizziness. Care is necessary in hypotensive states.

oxprenolol A beta-adrenoceptor blocking agent with the actions, uses and side-effects of propranolol. It also has anxiolytic properties, and may reduce the symptoms of transient stress such as tremor and palpitations. *Dose:* 60–480mg daily.

oxybuprocaine A local anaesthetic for ophthalmic use, including tonometry, as a 0.4% solution.

oxybutynin An anticholinergic antispasmodic that promotes relaxation of the detrusor muscle of the bladder. Dose in urinary incontinence 10–20mg daily; 10mg daily for children with neurogenic bladder instability. Side-effects are those of anticholinergic drugs generally.

†**oxycodone** A powerful narcotic analgesic with a prolonged action. Used as suppositories of 30mg.

oxymetazoline A long-acting nasal decongestant. Used as 0.05% drops twice a day.

oxymetholone A steroid related to testosterone. In oxymetholone, and in related steroids, the anabolic action of testosterone has been largely separated from the androgen or virilizing action. It is used mainly in aplastic and refractory anaemias, and in malignancy when bone marrow activity is depressed. *Dose:* 2–3mg/kg daily, but treatment for some months may be required. Some virilizing side-effects in female patients and children may occur with high doses. Contra-indicated in prostatic carcinoma, and care is necessary in renal, hepatic and cardiac insufficiency.

oxypertine A tranquillizer with a chlorpromazine-like action, and used in anxiety neuroses, psychoses and schizophrenic states. *Dose:* 30–60mg daily in anxiety states; up to 300mg daily in schizophrenia. In higher doses it may cause nausea, dizziness and drowsiness.

oxyphenbutazone A non-steroidal anti-inflammatory agent that is too toxic for systemic use, but has some value as a 10% ointment for inflamed conditions of the eye.

oxytetracycline See tetracycline.

oxytocin The oxytocic fraction of pituitary extract, but also made synthetically. Used for the induction and maintenance of labour, and to control post-partum haemorrhage, either alone or in association with ergometrine. *Dose:* 1–3 milli-units/ min by intravenous infusion. Excessive doses may cause severe uterine contractions with the risk of fetal asphyxiation.

P

padimate An absorbent of some of the erythema-producing ultraviolet light rays. It is used as a sunscreen as a 2.5% solution, but frequent application is necessary.

pamidronate See disodium pamidronate.

pancreatin A preparation containing the pancreatic enzymes, trypsin, lipase and amylase. It is used to aid the digestion of fats, proteins and carbohydrates in cystic fibrosis and pancreatitis. The action is inhibited by gastric acid, and pre-dosing with antacids and a drug of the cimetidine type increases the response. *Dose:* 2–4g with each meal.

pancuronium A non-depolarizing or competitive muscle relaxant similar to tubocurarine, but with the advantage that it has little histamine-releasing or cardiovascular action. *Dose:* 50–100μg/kg intravenously initially with supplementary doses of 10–20μg/kg as required.

papaveretum A preparation of the alkaloids of opium, containing approximately 50% of morphine. Used mainly by injection, often in association with hyoscine (scopolamine) for premedication. *Dose:* 10–20mg. It is now considered that noscopine, present in papaveretum, may possibly be genotoxic, and papaveretum is now contra-indicated in women of child-bearing age.

papaverine One of the alkaloids of opium. It has little analgesic action, and has been used mainly as a smooth muscle relaxant in peripheral vascular diseases, spasm and asthma. *Dose:* 60–300mg orally, 30–100mg by injection. It has caused cardiac arrhythmias.

paracetamol A widely used mild analgesic with few side-effects. It differs from aspirin in the absence of any anti-inflammatory action. *Dose:* 2–4g daily. Paediatric suppositories of 125mg are available. Overdose may cause severe liver damage (see acetylcysteine).

paraffin A generic name for hydrocarbon mixtures. Soft paraffin is the common ointment base; liquid paraffin is a lubricant laxative. Hard paraffin is used in the wax bath treatment of rheumatic conditions.

paraformaldehyde A solid form of formaldehyde, formerly used for disinfecting rooms, etc., by vaporization.

paraldehyde A colourless liquid with a strong characteristic odour. It is a rapid-acting sedative similar in effect to chloral, but causes less respiratory depression. It is also used in status asthmaticus. It may be given orally as a mixture, or by deep intramuscular injection. Occasionally given rectally after dilution with arachis oil. *Dose:* 5–10ml orally or by injection (using a *glass* syringe), 15–30ml rectally. Discoloured paraldehyde must *NOT* be used.

parathyroid The small glands associated with the thyroid, controlling calcium metabolism. Damage or loss of function results in hypocalcaemic tetany, which can be relieved by calcium gluconate injections, followed by oral calciferol.

paroxetine A selective inhibitor of serotonin uptake in the central nervous system, and indicated in the treatment of depression. *Dose:* 20mg daily, initially in the morning, with food, slowly increased as required to 50mg daily. It should not be given with any other drug likely to increase serotonin uptake. Side-effects are nausea, drowsiness and insomnia. See page 185.

pemoline A central nervous stimulant of medium potency. Useful in fatigue and reactive depression. Paradoxically, sometimes of value in hyperactive children. *Dose:* 40–120mg daily. Hallucinations may be a side-effect.

penbuterol A beta-adrenoceptor blocking agent with the actions and uses of propranolol, but available only as a mixed product with frusemide.

penicillamine A breakdown product of penicillin, which has the power of combining with certain metals to form a water-soluble, non-toxic complex that is excreted in the urine. It is used in Wilson's disease, which is due to the retention of copper in the body, in poisoning by lead and mercury, in chronic active hepatitis (after the condition has been controlled), in cystinuria, and in severe rheumatoid arthritis in which it has an action similar to that of gold. *Dose:* in Wilson's disease, 1.5–2g daily before food for some months. In chronic hepatitis, 500mg daily is given initially, slowly increased over some weeks to 1.25g daily. In rheumatoid arthritis, 125–250mg daily initially, before food, slowly increased at monthly intervals with maintenance doses of 500–750mg daily. Patients should be warned that the response in rheumatoid arthritis is slow. In cystinuria, 1–3g daily with adequate fluids, adjusted later to maintain the urinary cystine level below 200mg/l. In heavy metal poisoning, 0.5–2g daily. Side-effects include nausea, loss of taste, rash and thrombocytopenia. Blood counts during treatment are essential. A late onset rash may require cessation of treatment. See page 214.

penicillin, benzyl pencillin, penicillin G The first of the antibiotics. It is well tolerated and is widely used in the treatment of infections due to Gram-positive organisms and the spirochaetes of syphilis and yaws. It acts by preventing the development of the bacterial cell wall, but some groups of organisms vary widely in the degree of sensitivity, and it is inactivated by pencillinase-producing organisms. Penicillin is inactive orally, and so is given by intramuscular injection, but as it is rapidly excreted the action is relatively brief. Derivatives such as procaine-penicillin have a longer action (penicillin V is an orally active derivative). *Dose:* 600mg–2.4g daily. In severe infections up to 24g daily by intravenous infusion may be given. The main side-effect is hypersensitivity, and sensitivity to one penicillin extends to any other penicillins, and may also include sensitivity to the related cephalosporins. High doses of penicillin, especially in patients with renal insufficiency, may occasionally cause cerebral irritation and encephalopathy. Methicillin, cloxacillin and amoxycillin, are derivatives of penicillin active against resistant staphylococci; ampicillin has a wide range of activity against Gram-positive and Gram-negative organisms; carbenicillin, piperacillin and ticarcillin are active against *Pseudomonas aeruginosa*.

pentaerythritol tetranitrate A vasodilator with properties resembling those of glyceryl trinitrate, but with a more prolonged action. Used mainly in the prophylaxis of angina, as side-effects are relatively infrequent. *Dose:* 60–240mg daily.

pentamidine A synthetic drug used in the treatment of *Pneumocystis carinii* pneumonia in AIDS and other immunocompromised patients, as an alternative to co-trimoxazole. *Dose:* 4mg/kg daily by intravenous infusion for 14 days or more, or by inhalation of a nebulized solution. Other dosage schemes are used in the treatment of trypanosomiasis and leishmaniasis. Severe reactions, particularly hypotension, may occur, and pentamidine should be used only under expert supervision.

†**pentazocine** A powerful analgesic of the morphine type, but less likely to cause addition, although dependence may occur with long treatment. *Dose:* 100–400mg daily after food, up to 360mg daily by injection. Suppositories of 50mg are available. Hallucinations are an occasional side-effect. It should be avoided after myocardial infarction as it may increase the cardiac load. Other side-effects include dizziness, nausea, headache, tachycardia and rash. It should be avoided in opioid-dependent patients.

peppermint oil Aromatic carminative. Used as peppermint water as a flavouring agent in mixtures.

pericyazine A tranquillizer of the chlorpromazine type with similar uses and side-effects. It is used mainly in schizophrenia and severe anxiety states. *Dose:* 10–25mg or more, according to need.

pergolide A dopamine agonist with a stimulating action on both D_1 and D_2 receptors. It is used in the auxillary treatment of parkinsonism, and combined treatment may permit a reduction in dose of levodopa and its side-effects. *Dose:* 100μg daily initially, slowly increased at 3-day intervals according to response, with care taken to avoid hypotensive side-effects. Other side-effects include nausea, diarrhoea, confusion and hallucinations. See page 210.

perindopril A long-acting ACE inhibitor used in the control of essential and renovascular hypertension not responding to other drugs. Initially a single daily dose of 2mg (before food) is given, subsequently adjusted up to a maximum of 8mg daily. Diuretic therapy should first be withdrawn for 2–3 days, and renal function should be assessed before and during treatment. See page 199.

perphenazine A tranquillizer with the actions, uses and side-effects of chlorpromazine, but it is less sedating, and effective in lower doses. *Dose:* psychiatric and anti-emetic, 12–24mg daily. In severe vomiting 5–10mg by intramuscular injection. It is sometimes useful in the control of intractable hiccup.

†**pethidine** A synthetic analgesic with spasmolytic properties. Widely employed as an alternative to morphine for pre- and post-operative use. Of value in obstetrics as it has a less depressant action than morphine on the respiration. *Dose:* 300–900mg daily; by subcutaneous or intramuscular injection doses of 25–100mg at intervals according to need. Occasionally pet-

hidine is given by slow intravenous injection in doses of 25–50mg. *Dose:* as a supplementary analgesic in general anaesthesia, 10–25mg intravenously. Side-effects include dizziness, nausea and palpitations.

†**phenazocine** A synthetic morphine-like analgesic, with similar properties and uses, but with a more rapid and prolonged action. It is of value in biliary colic, as it is less likely to cause a rise in biliary pressure. *Dose:* 20–30mg daily, orally or sublingually, although single doses as high as 20mg are sometimes given. The side-effects are similar to those of morphine and related drugs, but sedation and the risk of dependence is less.

phenelzine A monoamine oxidase inhibitor, used in the treatment of depression. Its action may be linked with a rise in the amount of noradrenaline and other amines in the brain. *Dose:* 45–60mg daily, according to need and response. It has many side-effects, including dizziness, dry mouth and blurred vision. Very severe hypertension has been precipitated by some foods, notably cheese. Care is necessary in cardiovascular disease and epilepsy. It may also potentiate the action of other drugs on the central nervous system. See page 185.

phenethicillin A penicillin-derivative that is effective orally, giving blood levels comparable with those following injection of penicillin. Indicated in infections due to penicillin-sensitive organisms and in some skin and soft tissue infections. *Dose:* 1g daily, at least 30 min before food.

phenindamine An antihistamine of medium potency. It differs from most antihistamines in having a mild central stimulant action, and so rarely causes drowsiness. *Dose:* 75–200mg daily.

phenindione An orally active anticoagulant used in the control of deep-vein thrombosis. *Dose:* 200–300mg initially; maintenance, 25–100mg daily, depending on laboratory reports of the prothrombin time. Side-effects include hypersensitivity reactions and haemorrhage. Patients should be warned that the drug may colour the urine. Phenindione has now been largely replaced by warfarin.

pheniramine An antihistamine similar to, but less potent than chlorpheniramine. *Dose:* 150mg daily.

†**phenobarbitone** A powerful sedative, hypnotic and anticonvulsant drug. It is mainly of value in epilepsy, as it is effective in most types of seizure except petit mal (absence seizures). *Dose:* 60–180mg daily, at night, adjus-

ted to need and response. In severe conditions, doses of 50–200mg may be given by intramuscular or intravenous injection. Side-effects include drowsiness and skin reactions. In the elderly it may cause confusion, and paradoxically, it may give rise to hyperkinesia in some children.

phenol Once widely used as a general antiseptic. Weak solutions relieve itching, and phenol is present in Calamine Lotion. A 5% solution in almond oil is used for the injection treatment of haemorrhoids.

phenolphthalein A synthetic laxative. It is partly excreted in the bile, and may have an extended action by being reabsorbed via the entero-hepatic circulation. It is sometimes given with emulsion of liquid paraffin. *Dose:* 50–100mg daily. It may occasionally cause a rash, and its use has declined.

phenolsulphonphthalein A red compound used by i.v. injection in doses of 6mg as a test of renal function. In health, at least 50% of the test dose will be excreted in the urine 1 hr after the injection.

†**phenoperidine** A narcotic analgesic, often used in association with droperidol in neuroleptanalgesia. It is also used as a supplementary analgesic in general anaesthesia. *Dose:* 0.5–1mg IV with subsequent doses as required. It may cause respiratory depression, which can be controlled by doxapram or naloxone.

phenoxybenzamine An alpha-adrenoceptor blocking agent used in Raynaud's disease, vasospasm, and in the severe, episodic hypertension associated with phaeochromocytoma. *Dose:* orally and by injection, 10–20mg according to need and response. Side-effects include dizziness and tachycardia.

phenoxymethylpenicillin An orally active, acid-stable penicillin, also known as penicillin V. It is used mainly in respiratory infections in children; in tonsillitis, and to supplement injection treatment. It is not suitable for use in severe infections. *Dose:* 1–2g daily, before food.

phentermine An appetite depressant given in the short-term treatment of obesity. *Dose:*15–30mg before breakfast. See diethylpropion.

phentolamine An alpha-adrenoceptor blocking agent that can temporarily reverse the vascoconstrictive action of adrenaline and noradrenaline. It is used mainly in the diagnosis and control of phaeochromocytoma, and during surgical removal of the tumour. It is also useful in the hypertensive crises that may follow the abrupt withdrawal of clonidine, and in the control of acute ventricular failure. *Dose:* 5–10mg intravenously, repeated as required; or 5–60mg by intravenous infusion. Side-effects are tachycardia, hypotension, dizziness, nausea and diarrhoea.

phenylbutazone A powerful non-steroidal anti-inflammatory agent, formerly used in treatment of rheumatic and arthritic conditions. Because of blood dyscrasias, which may occur suddenly and fluid retention that may precipitate cardiac failure, the drug is now used only for the treatment of ankylosing spondylitis under hospital supervision. *Dose:* 400–600mg daily.

phenylephrine A vasoconstrictor similar to adrenaline, but less toxic. Given in acute hypotensive states. *Dose:* 5mg by intramuscular injection, or 100–500μg by slow intravenous injection. Sometimes valuable in paroxysmal atrial tachycardia. It is also used locally as 1:400 solution as nasal decongestive, and as eye-drops, 0.1–10%.

phenylmercuric nitrate A mercurial antibacterial and antifungal agent. Once used in antifungal creams and as a preservative in injections.

phenylpropanolamine A sympathomimetic agent used with other drugs in preparations for the symptomatic relief of nasal congestion.

phenytoin An anticonvulsant used in all forms of epilepsy with the exception of petit mal (absence seizures). It has little hypnotic effect and combined treatment with phenobarbitone may evoke the best response. *Dose:* 150–600mg daily. In status epilepticus it is given under ECG control in doses of 10–15mg/kg by slow intravenous injection. It is also given to control ventricular tachycardias, in doses of 3.5–5mg/kg by slow intravenous injection via a caval catheter. The side-effects of extended treatment are numerous, and include rash, dizziness, blood dyscrasias, hirsutism and gingival hypertrophy. See page 192.

pholcodine A cough centre depressant resembling codeine, but it lacks any analgesic properties. It is present in a range of products used for the relief of useless cough, and has the advantage over codeine of not causing constipation. *Dose:* 10–60mg daily.

physostigmine A plant alkaloid, also known as eserine, used as a miotic (0.25–1%) to counteract the effects of atropine, and in the treatment of glaucoma, often in association with pilocarpine. Solutions may turn pink on storage.

phthalylsulphathiazole A poorly absorbed sulphonamide once used in infective diarrhoea, but such use is no longer recommended.

phytomenadione Vitamin K_1. The form of vitamin K used in the prophylaxis and treatment of neonatal haemorrhage due to vitamin K deficiency. *Dose:* 1mg by intramuscular injection. It is also of value in the haemorrhage due to overdose of oral anticoagulants. *Dose:* 10–40mg by slow i.v. injection. Over-rapid injection may cause cyanosis and peripheral vascular collapse. In less severe conditions, 10–20mg orally, according to the base-line prothrombin time.

pilocarpine A plant alkaloid with a miotic action similar to, but less intense than, that of physostigmine. It is used in glaucoma as eye-drops of 0.5–4%, three to six times a day.

pimozide A tranquillizer with the actions and uses of chlorpromazine. It is used mainly in the treatment of schizophrenia, as it reduces the delusions without causing drowsiness. *Dose:* 20mg daily initially, adjusted up to a maximum of 60mg daily, with maintenance doses according to response. Similar doses are given in mania and psychomotor agitation. The side-effects are similar to those of chlorpromazine, but pimozide is less sedating. See page 216.

pindolol A beta-receptor blocking agent, with actions and uses similar to those of propranolol. Less likely to cause bronchospasm. *Dose:* 7.5–45mg daily.

pipenzolate An anticholinergic agent with some atropine-like antispasmodic properties. Used in peptic ulcer, irritable bowel syndrome and colic. *Dose:* 5mg before meals, and 5–10mg at night.

piperacillin A semi-synthetic penicillin with a wide range of activity that extends to *Pseudomonas* and anaerobes. It can be used in association with other antibiotics in life-threatening and multiple infections. *Dose:* in severe infections, 200–300mg/kg daily by i.m. or slow i.v. injection or infusion, increased in life-threatening infections up 16g daily. In less severe infections, 100–150mg/kg i.m. daily, with a maximum single dose of 2g. Piperacillin is not active orally.

piperazine An effective anthelmintic against threadworms and roundworms. *Dose:* 2–4 years, 750mg; 5–12 years, 1.5g; in children over 12 years and in adults, 2g; as a single daily dose for 7 days, repeated if necessary after 1 week. For roundworm, a single dose of 4g is given, but as the worms are narcotized, and not killed, a purgative is necessary to ensure expulsion. Side-effects are nausea, diarrhoea and occasional dizziness. Care is necessary in renal impairment, epilepsy and psychiatric conditions.

pipothiazine A chlorpromazine-like drug, with similar uses and side-effects, but given mainly as a depot preparation for the maintenance treatment of schizophrenia. *Dose:* (after a test dose of 25mg) 50–100mg by deep intramuscular injection every 4 weeks, increased if necessary up to a maximum of 200mg per dose.

pirbuterol A sympathomimetic drug with a selective action on beta$_2$ receptors, similar to salbutamol, thus causing bronchodilatation with little cardiac side-effects. Prophylactic oral *dose:* 30–60mg daily, or as aerosol inhalation 200–400μg (1–2 puffs). For maintenance treatment, and in severe bronchospasm, up to 12 puffs daily may be needed. See page 177. Care is necessary in cardiac disease and thyrotoxicosis.

pirenzepine A selective inhibitor of the acid- and pepsin-producing cells of the gastric mucosa. It reduces the secretion of gastric acid and pepsin without the side-effects of anticholinergic drugs, and is of value in the treatment of peptic ulcer. *Dose:* 50mg twice a day before meals for 4–6 weeks. In resistant conditions it may be given with drugs of the cimetidine type. Occasional side-effects are dryness of the mouth and visual disturbances.

piretanide A loop diuretic for use in mild hypertension. *Dose:* 6–12mg daily, in the morning. Care is necessary in prostatic hypertrophy, liver disease or any electrolyte imbalance. Side-effects include gastrointestinal disturbance and allergic reactions. Excess fluid loss in the elderly may cause circulatory disturbance.

piroxicam A non-steroidal anti-inflammatory agent with an extended action, and used in arthritis, spondylitis, gout and musculoskeletal disorders. *Dose:* 20–30mg daily; up to 40mg daily in gout and other acute conditions. It is also used for local application as a 3% gel. As with related drugs, side-effects include gastrointestinal disturbances of varying severity, especially with higher doses.

pituitary extract An aqueous extract of the posterior lobe of the pituitary gland. It has been used as an antidiuretic in diabetes insipidus, but analogues such as desmopressin are now preferred.

pivampicillin A derivative of ampicillin, with similar

actions and uses. Is hydrolysed to ampicillin after absorption, but gives higher blood levels. Much is excreted in the urine, so it is of value in urinary infections. *Dose:* 1–2g daily.

pivmecillinam An orally active form of mecillinam. Used mainly in urinary infections especially those due to enterobacteria such as *E.coli*. *Dose:* 800mg–2.4g daily.

pizotifen A serotonin antagonist used in the prophylaxis of migraine, and vascular headache. *Dose:* 1.5–3mg daily. Side-effects include drowsiness, nausea, dizziness and weight gain.

plicamycin A cytotoxic agent, also known as mithramycin, now used only to control the hypercalcaemia associated with malignancy. *Dose:* 25μg/kg by intravenous infusion daily for 3–4 days, but toxicity usually limits treatment, and other agents are often preferred. See disodium etidronate.

podophyllum resin A plant extract used topically as a paint (5–25% in alcohol) for anogenital and plantar warts. It is very irritant to normal tissues, and its use requires care.

poldine A synthetic atropine-like drug used in hyperacidity, gastric ulcer and other conditions associated with smooth muscle spasm. *Dose:* 10–30mg daily. Side-effects are those of the anticholinergic drugs generally.

polygeline A modified gelatin, used with sodium chloride and other electrolytes as a blood volume expander. *Dose:* 500–1000ml by i.v. infusion.

polymyxin B An antibiotic used in infections due to *Ps. aeruginosa* and other Gram-negative bacteria. Kidney damage limit its systemic value, and less toxic antibiotics such as carbenicillin and gentamicin are now preferred . *Dose:* up to 25 000 units/kg daily by slow i.v. infusion. Also used for topical application.

polymyxin E See colistin.

polystyrene resin An ion-exchange resin for the removal of potassium in conditions associated with hyperkalaemia, as in oliguria and anuria. *Dose:* 15g three or four times a day according to the plasma level of potassium. When the drug is not tolerated orally, 30g daily as a suspension may be given per rectum. Care is required in renal or hepatic impairment.

polythiazide A potent diuretic with the actions, uses and side-effects of the thiazide diuretics but effective in the low dose of 1–4mg daily.

potassium One of the most important ions of the body, mainly present in intracellular fluid. Many diuretics increase loss of potassium as well as sodium; with extended treatment the potassium balance may be disturbed, with acute muscle weakness, cardiac arrhythmias, and an increased sensitivity to digitalis. Potassium loss can be treated with potassium chloride orally (often as Slow-K, but may cause peptic ulceration), or by effervescent potassium tablets. Mixed diuretic and potassium products are not entirely satisfactory. In acute potassium deficiency, various potassium-containing intravenous solutions are available, but dose and rate of administration require care, as in excess, potassium can cause cardiac arrest. Intravenous solutions should not contain more than 3.2g/litre of potassium chloride.

potassium citrate A diuretic useful in cystitis and other inflammatory conditions of the urinary tract to produce alkalization of the urine. It is also given in gout to increase the excretion of uric acid, and during sulphonamide therapy to prevent crystalluria. *Dose:* 9–24g daily.

potassium iodide It reduces the viscosity of bronchial mucus, and has been used as an expectorant; it has been used in the prophylaxis and treatment of simple goitre which is due to a deficiency of iodide. It has also been given pre-operatively in thyrotoxicosis, as it alters the texture of the gland, and facilitates surgery. *Dose:* as an expectorant, 250–500mg; in thyrotoxicosis, 150mg daily.

potassium permanganate Purple crystals, soluble in water. A powerful oxidizing and deodorizing agent used 1:1000 as lotion, 1:10 000 to 1:5000 as mouthwash, douche, bladder washout and bath.

povidone-iodine A complex of iodine with an organic carrier such as povidone is termed an iodophore. When applied to the skin, iodophores slowly release iodine, and have an extended antiseptic action. Used for local application to the skin and mucous membranes as solution containing the equivalent of 0.75%–1% of iodine.

pralidoxime A reactivator of cholinesterase. Organophosphorus insecticides inhibit that enzyme, and poisoning by such insecticides is an occupational hazard. Their toxicity can be reversed in part by the injection of 2mg atropine, but the enzyme can be reactivated by the intravenous injection of 1g pralidoxime. It is effective only if given within 24 hrs of exposure to the insecticide.

pravastatin A cholesterol lowering agent with the specific enzyme-inhibiting properties of simvastatin, and used in primary hypercholesterolaemia not responding to other drugs. It is said to have an action largely limited to the liver, so extrahepatic side-effects are correspondingly reduced. *Dose:* 10–40mg daily as a single dose. Side-effects include myalgia, rash and gastrointestinal disturbances. See page 197.

prazinquantel A schistosomicide of low toxicity, effective against *Schistosoma haematobium*, *S. mansoni* and *S. japonicum.* It is also active against tapeworm. *Dose:* 40mg/kg as a single oral dose. It is well tolerated.

prazosin An alpha-adrenoceptor blocking agent and vasodilator. It is used in the treatment of hypertension and congestive heart failure. *Dose:* 1mg daily initially, increased as required up to a maximum of 20mg daily. The initial dose may cause marked hypotension, and it should be taken at night, in bed. Prazocin is also given in benign prostatic hypertrophy in maintenance doses of 4mg daily. Side-effects are drowsiness, nausea and postural hypotension.

prednisolone A glucocorticosteroid with the actions and uses of hydrocortisone, but effective in much lower doses. It is often the preferred drug for oral use, and is given in a wide range of conditions, including asthma, severe allergic reactions, rheumatoid arthritis and collagen disorders, and inflammatory skin conditions. Prednisolone is also of value in leukaemia, ulcerative colitis, the nephrotic syndrome, pemphigus, sarcoidosis, myasthenia gravis, haemolytic anaemia, agranulocytosis and other blood dyscrasias. Large doses are given in the immunosuppressive control of transplant surgery. The dose varies with the nature of the condition being treated, and its severity, and in every case the lowest dose required to evoke an adequate response should be used, after which the dose should be reduced in stages. *Dose:* in rheumatoid arthritis, 7.5–10mg daily initially; other conditions may require doses up to 100mg daily. Dose by intramuscular injection 25–100mg once or twice a week. As a retention enema, 20mg to relieve the inflammation of colitis and Crohn's disease; as eye-drops and ear-drops, 0.5% solution. The side-effects are those of the corticosteroids generally, and include salt and water retention, hypertension, muscle weakness and peptic ulcer.

prednisone A glucocorticosteroid that is converted to

prednisolone in the body, and so has the actions and uses of that drug.

prilocaine A local anaesthetic with the actions, uses and side-effects of lignocaine.

primaquine An antimalarial drug used mainly to prevent a relapse of benign tertian malaria after treatment with chloroquine, as it kills the malarial parasites that may still be present in the liver. *Dose:* 15mg daily, for 2–3 weeks after chloroquine treatment. Side-effects are nausea and abdominal pain.

primidone An anticonvulsant used in the treatment of grand mal and psychomotor epilepsy, but some cases of petit mal also respond. *Dose:* 125mg daily initially, slowly increased as required up to a maximum of 1.5g daily. Side-effects include drowsiness, nausea, blurred vision and rash.

probenecid An orally active compound that increases the excretion of uric acid, and so is useful in the treatment of gout and hyperuricaemia. *Dose:* 0.5–2g daily. An adequate fluid intake and an alkaline urine are necessary for the best response. Probenecid also has the property of delaying the excretion of penicillin and some cephalosporins, and is given in doses of 2g daily to raise the plasma level of those antibiotics. Side-effects include occasional nausea, flushing and dizziness.

probucol A plasma-cholesterol regulating agent used in some forms of hyperlipidaemia. *Dose:* 1g daily. Side-effects are nausea, flatulence and diarrhoea.

procainamide A procaine derivative occasionally of value in the treatment of ventricular arrhythmias. *Dose:* up to 50mg/kg daily. It is also given by slow intravenous injection under ECG control in doses of 25–50mg/minute up to a maximum of 1g. Side-effects are gastrointestinal disturbances, fever and rash.

procaine A local anaesthetic now largely replaced by lignocaine.

procaine penicillin An old form of long-acting penicillin given together with penicillin G to obtain a high initial blood level. It is now used mainly in early syphilis. *Dose:* 900mg daily for 10 days.

procarbazine A cytotoxic drug used mainly as part of a multidrug treatment of Hodgkin's disease. It is also used to treat other lymphomas, as well as solid tumours no longer responding to other therapy. *Dose:* 50mg initially, increasing to a maximum of 300mg daily. Side-effects include nausea, anorexia and bone marrow depression. Alcohol may cause a disulfiram reaction, and cheese should be avoided.

prochlorperazine A tranquillizer with the actions, uses and side-effects of chlorpromazine. *Dose:* in schizophrenia, 75–100mg daily; in severe anxiety, 10–40mg daily. In severe nausea and vomiting, 20mg orally, or 12.5mg by deep intramuscular injection. It is also used as suppositories of 25mg.

procyclidine A spasmolytic drug similar to benzhexol, used mainly in the treatment of parkinsonism. Reduces rigidity more than tremor. *Dose:* 7.5–30mg daily. In acute states it is given by intramuscular injection in doses of 5–10mg, or 5mg doses intravenously.

progesterone The hormone of the corpus luteum, responsible for the preparation of the uterus to receive a fertilized ovum. It is used in dysfunctional uterine bleeding and in the premenstrual syndrome. *Dose:* 200–400mg daily *per vagina* on a cyclic basis or by deep intramuscular injection in doses of 5–10mg for 5–10 days. See dydrogesterone and norethisterone.

proguanil hydrochloride A synthetic antimalarial of high potency and low toxicity, used in the prophylaxis and suppressive treatment of malaria. *Dose:* 100–200mg daily, and continued for 6 weeks after leaving the infected area.

prolintane A weak central stimulant, present in some mixed vitamin products used in debility.

promazine A tranquillizer with the actions, uses, and side-effects of chlorpromazine, but less potent. It is used mainly to control agitation in the elderly, and in other minor conditions of psychiatric disturbance. *Dose:* 50–800mg daily, adjusted to need and response; by injection, 25–50mg.

promethazine A long-acting antihistamine with sedative properties. It is used for the relief of a wide range of allergic conditions; in mild insomnia and for pre-operative sedation. It is also of value as an anti-emetic in the prophylaxis and treatment of travel sickness, vertigo, and drug-induced nausea. *Dose:* 25–75mg daily; 25–50mg by deep intramuscular injection. In anaphylaxis, sometimes given by slow intravenous injection in doses up to 100mg to supplement previously injected adrenaline. The side-effects are those of the antihistamines generally.

propafenone An anti-arrhythmic agent of the lignocaine type, used in the prophylaxis and treatment of ventricular arrhythmias.

Dose: under ECG control 450mg daily initially, increased at 3-day intervals up to a maximum of 900mg daily. Side-effects are dizziness, gastro-intestinal disturbances, and postural hypotension.

propantheline An anticholinergic agent used as a spasmolytic in gastrointestinal disorders, in urinary frequency associated with bladder neck weakness, and in nocturnal enuresis. *Dose:* 45–120mg daily. Side-effects include dryness of the mouth and blurred vision.

propofol A non-irritant short-acting i.v. anaesthetic for smooth induction and maintenance of general anaesthesia for up to 1 hr. *Dose:* 2–2.5mg/kg initially, followed by supplementary doses of 0.1–0.2mg/kg/min as required but some local pain may occur. Side-effects include mild hypotension, transient apnoea and bradycardia. Recovery is normally rapid and uneventful but delayed recovery, convulsions and anaphylaxis have been reported. Care is necessary in cardiovascular, respiratory or renal impairment.

propranolol A beta-adrenoceptor blocking agent that reduces the cardiac response to circulating adrenaline. It reduces the load on the heart during exercise and stress, and is used in the treatment of angina, coronary insufficiency, cardiac arrhythmias, hypertension, and after myocardial infarction. It also ameliorates the tremor and palpitation of transient anxiety and stress, and is useful in the prophylactic treatment of migraine. *Dose:* 160–320mg daily according to need. In arrhythmias and thyrotoxic crisis, propranolol is given by slow intravenous injection in doses of 1mg, repeated up to a maximum of 10mg. Side-effects are bradycardia, bronchospasm and gastro-intestinal disturbances. Care is necessary in renal and hepatic deficiency; asthma is a contra-indication.

propylthiouracil A thyroid inhibitor occasionally used as an alternative to carbimazole in hyperthyroidism. *Dose:* 300–450mg daily.

prostacyclin Epoprostenol.

prostaglandin A generic term applied to a series of closely related hormone-like fatty acid derivatives, originally extracted from prostate gland, but now prepared synthetically. Prostaglandins are widely distributed in animal tissues, and have a complex and varying range of biological activity. Thus they may have a smooth muscle stimulating or relaxant action, pressor, vasodilator, inflammatory or other properties. There is evidence that the anti-inflammatory action of aspirin and related drugs may be due to an inhibition of prostaglandin synthesis. There are four main groups of prostaglandins (PGA, PGB, PGE and PGF) which can be further subdivided. PGE_2, and PGF_2, have been given by intravenous infusion in the induction of labour and in the termination of pregnancy, and an oral form is available as dinoprostone. Alprostadil (PGE_1) is used to maintain the patency of the ductus arteriosus in some neonates.

protamine sulphate A simple protein obtained from fish sperm. It neutralizes the anticoagulant effect of heparin, and it is used in controlling the haemorrhage that may occur during heparin therapy. *Dose:* 1% solution intravenously according to need; 1mg will neutralize 80–100 units of heparin.

prothionamide An antitubercular drug, used in resistant tuberculosis, and when first-choice drugs are not tolerated. It is also used in the treatment of leprosy. *Dose:* 0.5–1g daily. Side-effects are gastrointestinal disturbances, peripheral neuritis, vertigo and photophobia.

protirelin The thyrotrophin-releasing hormone (TRH) of the hypothalamus. It is used in the diagnosis of hyperthyroidism as a single intravenous dose of 200μg. It normally induces a rapid rise in the plasma levels of thyrotrophin, but in thyrotoxicosis that rise does not occur. Side-effects include nausea, flushing, a strange taste and urinary urgency.

protriptyline A tricyclic antidepressant with actions and uses similar to amitriptyline. It is used in depression associated with apathy, as it has some stimulant action. *Dose:* 15–60mg daily. Side-effects are cardiovascular disturbance, rash and photosensitivity.

proxymetacaine A local anaesthetic used as 0.5% drops in ophthalmology.

pseudoephedrine A drug very closely related to ephedrine, but said to have reduced central effects. Used mainly as a respiratory decongestant and occasionally in nocturnal enuresis. *Dose:* 60–240mg daily in adults, 60–120mg daily in children. May cause hallucinations in some children.

pyrantel A neuromuscular blocking agent used as a single-dose anthelmintic in threadworm, roundworm and hookworm infections. It paralyses susceptible worms, which are then excreted. *Dose:* 10mg/kg for adults and children over 6 months. Side-effects include gastrointestinal disturbance, dizziness, headache and rash.

pyrazinamide An antituberculous drug that is active against the intracellular and dividing forms of *M. tuberculosis*, and is most effective in the early stage of the disease. It penetrates the meninges, and is of value in tuberculous meningitis. *Dose:* 20–35mg/kg daily up to a maximum of 3g daily. Side-effects include fever, jaundice and hepatotoxicity. Liver function tests should be carried out before and during treatment.

pyridostigmine An anticholinesterase similar to neostigmine. It has a slower and more prolonged action that is useful in some cases of myasthenia gravis. *Dose:* 300–750mg daily. The side-effects are similar to those of neostigmine, but may be less severe.

pyridoxine (vitamin B_6) This vitamin plays an essential part in protein metabolism. Apart from its use in deficiency states, which are uncommon, pyridoxine has been used in isoniazid-induced neuropathy. *Dose:* 25–150mg daily; in some sideroblastic anaemias, up to 400mg daily.

pyrimethamine An antimalarial drug, used with dapsone as Maloprim or with sulphadoxine as Fansidar in the prophylaxis of chloroquine-resistant malaria. The use of these mixed products is not without risk, as they may have severe and sometimes fatal side-effects.

pyroxylin A nitrated cellulose used for the preparation of collodion.

Q

†quinalbarbitone sodium A short-acting barbiturate. Used in mild insomnia and anxiety states. *Dose:* 50–200mg.

quinapril An ACE inhibitor with the actions, use and side-effects of that group of drugs. *Dose:* in hypertension 5mg daily initially, slowly increased to 20–40mg as a single daily dose. See ACE inhibitors, and page 199.

quinidine An alkaloid of cinchona, similar to quinine, that has been used in the preventive treatment of ventricular arrhythmias, but beta-blocking agents, are now preferred. *Dose:* (after a test dose of 200mg) 200–400mg three to four times a day. Side-effects are tinnitus, vertigo and confusion. Treatment should be stopped if response does not occur within 10 days.

quinine The principal alkaloid of cinchona bark. It was once used extensively in the treatment of malignant tertian malaria, and recently it has regained some of its value with the emergence of chloroquine-resistant malaria. *Dose:* 1.8g daily for 5 days; in serious infections it is given by intravenous infusion in doses of 10mg/kg for up to three doses, followed by oral therapy. Side-effects include tinnitus, nausea, rash and visual disturbances.

R

ramipril An ACE inhibitor with the general properties of such drugs. *Dose:* in mild hypertension 1.25mg daily, increased at intervals of 1–2 weeks up to a maximum of 10mg, given with food and adequate fluid. See page 199.

ranitidine A powerful and selective histamine H_2 antagonist of the cimetidine type, but with a longer action. It reduces the volume, acidity and pepsin content of gastric secretion, and is of value in peptic ulcer, reflux oesophagitis and similar conditions. *Dose:* 300mg daily for at least 4 weeks, maintenance doses, 150mg daily. In severe conditions, 50mg by intramuscular or slow intravenous injection repeated at intervals of 6–8 hrs. In suspected gastric ulcer, malignancy should be excluded before treatment is commenced. Ranitidine is well tolerated, and as it is not anti-androgenic, gynaecomastia is unlikely to be a side-effect. See cimetidine.

rauwolfia The dried roots of *Rauwolfia serpentina.* It has a central depressant action, but it is used mainly in the treatment of mild hypertension as the chief alkaloid reserpine.

razoxane A cytotoxic agent used in the treatment of leukaemias. *Dose:* 250mg or more daily under laboratory control. Side-effects are nausea, diarrhoea, skin reactions and myelosuppression.

remoxipride A selective dopamine D_2 receptor antagonist used in acute chronic schizophrenia and other psychoses. *Dose:* 300mg daily initially, increasing up to 600mg if required, with maintenance doses of 150–300mg daily. Capsules should be swallowed whole with water. Side-effects are nausea, headache and weight change. Extrapyramidal side-effects similar to but less severe than with haloperidol. See page 216.

reproterol A bronchodilator with the actions, uses and side-effects of salbutamol. *Dose:* 30–60mg daily; by aerosol inhalation, 0.5–1mg (1–2 puffs), repeated up to six times a day. Side-effects include tremor and mild tachycardia. See page 178.

reserpine The principal alkaloid of rauwolfia. It is used in mild hypertension, but a fall in blood pressure occurs only after continued treatment. *Dose:* 100–250μg daily. It may cause depression, nasal congestion and gastric disturbances, and more controllable drugs are now preferred.

resorcin A keratolytic agent used mainly as an ointment in acne, and as a hair lotion for removing dandruff. Myxoedema has been reported following the prolonged use of resorcin preparations.

retinol Vitamin A.

Rheomacrodex A dextran preparation used mainly to improve blood flow and prevent 'sludging' of red cells after injury. Useful in various types of peripheral ischaemia.

rhubarb The dried rhizome of various species of *Rheum*, from China and Tibet. Used occasionally as a mild purgative and in small doses as an astringent bitter.

riboflavine (vitamin B_2) An orange-yellow powder. It is part of the vitamin B complex, and is concerned with the oxidation of carbohydrates and amino acids. A deficiency causes several characteristic effects, including angular stomatitis and 'burning feet'. *Dose:* 1–10mg in deficiency states associated with restricted diets or poor absorption.

rifampicin An antibiotic now considered to be the first-choice drug in the treatment of tuberculosis, and is given together with isoniazid and pyrazinamide. *Dose:* 600mg before breakfast. It is also used with dapsone in the initial treatment of severe leprosy. Side-effects include gastrointestinal disturbances, rash, an influenza-like syndrome and hepatic reactions. Jaundice is a contra-indication. Patients should be warned that rifampicin gives a red colour to the urine, sputum and tears, and to soft contact lenses. It may decrease the response to oral anticoagulants such as warfarin, and the failure of oral contraceptives has also been reported in patients receiving rifampicin.

rimiterol A bronchodilator similar in actions and uses to salbutamol, but with a shorter duration of effect. It is largely free from any cardiac stimulant activity. Rimiterol is used mainly for the relief of bronchospasm in bronchitis, bronchial asthma and similar conditions. *Dose:* by aerosol inhalation, 200–600μg (1–3 puffs) up to a maximum of 8 puffs daily.

Ringer's solution An electrolyte replacement solution containing sodium chloride, potassium chloride and calcium chloride.

ritodrine A sympathomimetic

drug with a relaxant action on uterine muscle, and used to inhibit premature labour. *Dose:* 50μg/min initially by intravenous infusion, slowly increased up to 350μg/min, or 10mg by intramuscular injection and continued until the contractions have ceased; then orally up to 120mg daily to prevent relapse. Side-effects include tremor, nausea and hypotension.

Rose bengal A dye used as eye-drops (1%) to stain and detect devitalized conjunctival cells, and in the diagnosis of dry eye.

rosoxacin See acrosoxacin.

rubella vaccine A suspension of a live, attenuated strain of rubella virus. It is used for active immunization in girls of 10–14 years, and in seronegative women of childbearing age. *Dose:* 0.5ml by subcutaneous injection. It is contra-indicated in pregnancy, and pregnancy within 3 months of vaccination should be avoided.

S

saccharin An organic chemical widely used as a non-calorific substitute for sugar. Has been used by rapid intravenous injection (2.5g in 4ml) for arm–tongue circulation time.

salbutamol A selective $beta_2$-adrenoceptor stimulant. It is widely used to relieve bronchospasm in airway obstruction, including bronchial asthma and status asthmaticus, with the advantage of being largely free from cardiac side-effects. *Dose:* up to 16mg orally daily; by aerosol inhalation (in which patients should be carefully instructed) 100–200μg (1–2 puffs) up to four times a day; by subcutaneous or intramuscular injection 500μg as required; 250μg by intravenous injection. Salbutamol also relaxes uterine muscle, and is given in premature labour in doses of 10μg/min initially by intravenous infusion, increased to 45μg/min until contractions have ceased, when oral therapy may be given. Side-effects include tremor, headache, peripheral vasodilatation and tachycardia. Care is necessary in ischaemic heart disease, hypertension and hyperthyroidism. See page 177.

salcatonin A synthetic form of calcitonin, preferred for extended use, as it is less likely to provoke allergic reactions.

salicylic acid Has useful keratolytic and fungicidal properties. Used as ointment (2%) for skin conditions, and as ointments and plasters (up to 40%) for corns and warts.

salmeterol A salbutamol derivative for the long-term regular prophylaxis of asthma, bronchitis and other forms of obstructive airway disease. It is given in doses of 50μg twice daily, either from a metered dose aerosol or by a 'Diskhaler'. Salmeterol is well tolerated, but headache, tremor and tachycardia may occur with doses above 200μg daily. See page 177.

salsalate A long-acting mild analgesic of the aspirin type, but less likely to cause any gastric disturbance. *Dose:* 2–4g daily.

Savlon A mixture of cetrimide and chlorhexidine, widely used as an effective and non-irritant antiseptic.

scopolamine See hyoscine.

selegiline A selective enzyme inhibitor that prevents the inactivation of dopamine in the brain. It is used to supplement the action of levodopa in the treatment of parkinsonism, and combined use may give a smoother response, and permit a reduction in the dose of levodopa. *Dose:* 5–10mg daily. It may cause nausea and hypotension, and may possibly increase the side-effects of levodopa.

selenium sulphide Used as a shampoo in the treatment of dandruff. Prolonged use may cause alopecia.

senna The leaves and pods of *Cassia* sp., used as a purgative. Standardized preparations such as Senokot are now preferred.

serotonin A substance present in many body cells, which also acts as a neurotransmitter in the central nervous system. A reduction in brain serotonin levels may be associated with depression and the cranial vasodilation associated with migraine. (See page 204.) Some allergic reactions may also be linked with the action of serotonin on sensitized cells (see cyproheptadine).

sertraline An antidepressant that functions as an inhibitor of serotonin uptake. It is used both for the treatment of depression and the prevention of relapse. *Dose:* 50mg daily initially with food, increased at weekly intervals up to a maximum of 200mg daily. Not to be given with monoamine oxidase inhibitors. Side-effects are tremor and dryness of the mouth. See page 185.

silicones Synthetic water-repellent substances present in barrier creams and other skin protective products. Dimethicone is a silicone used as an anti-foaming agent in some antacid preparations.

silver nitrate Used mainly as silver nitrate sticks (caustic points) for cauterizing warts. It has also been used as a 0.5% lotion for suppurating lesions. It was once used prophylactically as eye-drops (0.1%) in the newborn, and is still used for that purpose in the USA.

silver sulphadiazine Sulphadiazine combined with silver. It is used topically as a 1% cream for its wide-range antibacterial properties in burns and infected skin conditions, especially when an extended action is required. It is active against *Pseudomonas aeruginosa* and other Gram-negative organisms.

simvastatin A new compound with a selective action on a specific enzyme concerned with the synthesis of cholesterol in the liver. It is used in the treatment of primary hypercholesterolaemia in patients not responding to other drugs. *Dose:* 10–40mg at night. Liver function tests should be carried out regularly, and eye examinations annually. Side-effects include gastro-intestinal disturbances. See page 197.

snake-bite antivenom A bite from an adder, the only poisonous snake indigenous to the UK can cause local pain and swelling as well as systemic effects such as colic and vomiting, but death from adder-bite is very rare. If the reaction to an adder bite is severe, Zagreb anti-venom, if available, should be given by intravenous infusion within 4 hrs of the bite.

soda-lime A mixture of calcium and sodium hydroxides, used in closed-circuit anaesthetic apparatus to remove carbon dioxide.

sodium acetrizoate An iodine compound used as a contrast agent in intravenous pyelography.

sodium acid phosphate An acid diuretic, given with hexamine. In full doses it acts as a saline purgative. *Dose:* 2–4g.

sodium aurothiomalate A gold compound used in the treatment of active rheumatoid arthritis. It is of no value in other forms of the disease, or where bone change has already occurred. *Dose:* 10mg by deep intramuscular injection weekly initially, slowly increased to 50mg weekly, and continued until a remission occurs, or until a total dose of 1g has been given. Blood and urine tests are essential after each injection. After remission, 20–50mg may be given every 2–4 weeks for many months. Side-effects are common, and include blood disorders, skin reactions, mouth ulcers and oedema, and may require withdrawal of the drug. It is contra-indicated in renal and hepatic disease, blood dyscrasias and hypertension. See auranofin and page 214.

sodium benzoate When given by injection, it is excreted as hippuric acid, and the rate of excretion is sometimes used as an indication of liver function.

sodium bicarbonate A widely used soluble antacid, often in association with less soluble antacids such as magnesium carbonate or trisilicate. *Dose:* 1–4g. In severe metabolic acidosis it is given by slow intravenous injection as an 8.4% solution. For alkalization of the urine, up to 3g orally 2 hrly with further 10g doses daily as required.

sodium calcium edetate A chelating or binding agent used in poisoning by lead and other heavy metals. *Dose:* 80mg/kg daily by intravenous infusion in glucose/saline solution. Nausea and cramp are side-effects, and care is necessary in renal impairment.

sodium cellulose phosphate An ion-exchange compound that binds with calcium in the intestines, and so reduces calcium absorption. It is used in the oral treatment of hypercalcaemia and renal stones, and as an adjunct to low-calcium diets. *Dose:* 15g daily. Diarrhoea is an occasional side-effect.

sodium clodronate A diphosphonate that suppresses bone resorption in the hypercalcaemia of malignancy, and promotes restoration of a clinically acceptable serum calcium level. *Dose:* 300mg by slow intravenous infusion daily for 3–5 days or more, followed by daily oral doses of 1.6g taken 2 hrs before or after food. Adequate fluids should be given. Side-effects are gastro-intestinal disturbances. Serum calcium and phosphate levels should be monitored. See disodium pamidronate.

sodium chloride An important constituent of blood and tissues. It is widely used by intravenous infusion as normal saline solution (0.9%), or as glucose-saline in the treatment of dehydration, shock and other conditions of sodium depletion. It is also useful when given orally as Sodium Chloride with Glucose Oral Powder (BNF) (after solution in water), for children with diarrhoea to offset any loss of salt. Its use as an emetic in the treatment of poisoning is no longer recommended. It is used externally as saline solution when a simple cleansing lotion is required.

sodium citrate An alkaline diuretic similar to potassium citrate and given for similar purposes. *Dose:* 1–4g. For citrating milk, 100mg to each feed may be used. A 3% solution is used by bladder irrigation for the dissolution of blood clots.

sodium cromoglycate An anti-allergic agent with a specific action and used for the prophylactic treatment of asthma by inhalation. It stabilizes mast cells and inhibits the release of histamine and other spasmogens that cause bronchospasm. *Dose:* by powder inhalation from a 'Spinhaler' 20mg up to eight times a day; by aerosol inhalation, 2mg (2 puffs), up to eight times a day. Dose in the treatment for food allergy associated with local inflammation, 800mg daily orally. It is also of value as eye-drops (2%) and eye-ointment (2%) in allergic conjunctivitis, and as nasal-drops or spray (2%) in the prophylaxis of allergic rhinitis. See page 177.

sodium fluoride The fluoride present in dentifrices used to reduce dental caries. It may also be given orally when more intensive treatment is required. *Dose:* 250–500μg daily.

sodium fusidate An antibiotic used mainly in penicillin-resistant staphylococcal infections, although a secondary antibiotic is often given as well to increase the response. It is useful in osteomyelitis and similar conditions as it penetrates into bone tissues. *Dose:* 2g daily. In severe infections, 1.5g daily by i.v. infusion. Side-effects include nausea, rash and jaundice. Liver function tests should be carried out during treatment.

sodium hypochlorite A weak solution of sodium hypochlorite containing 0.25% of available chlorine is used as eusol, for the cleansing of wounds and ulcers. The solution is unstable and should be freshly prepared. Its value has recently been questioned. Stronger, stabilized solutions are used for the general disinfection of surfaces contaminated with blood and other body fluids. Their use reduces the risk of transmission of hepatitis and other viral infections.

sodium ironedetate A soluble, non-irritant iron complex, available as a solution containing 27.5mg of iron per 5ml. It is used in the oral treatment of iron-deficiency anaemias, and is of value when other iron preparations are not tolerated. *Dose:* 15–30ml daily.

sodium lactate Has been used as M/6 solution, or as Hartmann's solution, by intravenous infusion for metabolic acidosis, but sodium bicarbonate is now preferred.

sodium nitrite A cyanide antidote. It is given as a 3% solution by intravenous injection of 10ml, followed by the slow injection of 25ml of sodium thiosulphate solution (50%). Early treatment is essential.

sodium nitroprusside A short-acting arteriovenous vasodilator, used in hypertensive crisis, and for controlled hypotension during anaesthesia. *Dose:* by i.v. infusion, 0.3–1μg/kg/min, the lower doses being used to obtain hypotension during surgery. It is also used in acute heart failure in doses of 10–15μg/min, increased as required to 200μg/min.

sodium perborate White powder soluble in water, with antiseptic and deodorant properties similar to hydrogen peroxide. A 2% solution is used as a mouthwash.

sodium phosphate A solution of sodium phosphate with sodium acid phosphate is sometimes used by enema as a laxative. These phosphates are also occasionally added to intravenous electrolyte solutions when a phosphate deficiency is present or suspected.

sodium picosulphate A synthetic laxative similar to bisacodyl, but with a slower action. *Dose:* 5–15mg at night.

sodium salicylate A soluble anti-inflammatory and analgesic agent. *Dose:* 2–10g daily. The side-effects are similar to those of aspirin.

sodium stibogluconate An organic antimony drug used in the treatment of visceral leishmaniasis or kala-azar. *Dose:* 10mg/kg daily by intramuscular or intravenous injection for 30 days. Side-effects include anorexia, vomiting, cough and substernal pain.

sodium tetradecyl sulphate A venous-occluding agent used in the compression-sclerosing treatment of varicose veins. *Dose:* 0.5–1ml at any one site, followed by compression bandaging for some weeks. The local irritant action of the drug brings about an occlusive venous fibrosis at the injection site. Extra-vascular injection may cause necrosis. Care is necessary in allergic subjects.

sodium thiosulphate A 50% solution is given by intravenous injection in cyanide poisoning. See sodium nitrite.

sodium valproate An anticonvulsant effective in most forms of epilepsy. *Dose:* 600mg daily in adults initially, increased if required up to a maximum of 2.5g daily. It may also be given by slow intravenous injection in doses of 400–800mg, followed by similar doses given by intravenous infusion. Liver function tests before and during treatment are essential. Severe side-effects such as vomiting, drowsiness or jaundice, require withdrawal of the drug, as does spontaneous bleeding or bruising. See page 192.

somatropin A form of human growth hormone obtained by biosynthesis. It is used to stimulate growth in hormone-deficient young patients whilst the epiphyses are still open. *Dose:* 0.07 units/kg daily by intramuscular or subcutaneous injection. Subcutaneous injection sites should be varied.

sorbide nitrate Isosorbide dinitrate.

sorbitol A saccharide that, after absorption, is converted in the liver almost entirely to laevulose. It has been used as a sugar-substitute in diabetes, and it is sometimes given by intravenous injection as a 50% solution to promote diuresis and to reduce cerebral oedema.

sotalol A beta-adrenergic blocking agent used in the treatment of hypertension, angina, cardiac arrhythmias and thyrotoxicosis. *Dose:* 100mg initially, increased as required; maintenance, 160–600mg daily. For prophylaxis after infarction, 320mg daily. In acute cardiac arrhythmias, 20–60mg by slow i.v. injection under ECG control. Care is necessary in heart block, asthma, hepatic and renal impairment.

spectinomycin An antibiotic used in the treatment of penicillin-resistant gonorrhoea. *Dose:* 2–4g by deep i.m. injection. Side-effects include nausea, dizziness and pruritus.

spironolactone An aldosterone antagonist which potentiates the action of thiazide and loop diuretics in some resistant conditions. It is of value in the oedema of liver cirrhosis, as well as in the nephrotic syndrome and congestive heart failure. *Dose:* 100mg daily up to a maximum dose of 400mg daily. Side-effects include drowsiness, gastrointestinal disturbances, gynaecomastia and an increased sensitivity to warfarin. The combined use of potassium-sparing diuretics or potassium supplements is contra-indicated.

stanozolol An anabolic steroid with actions and uses similar to those of nandrolone. *Dose:* 5mg daily. It also has fibrinolytic properties, and is used in lipodermatosclerosis (a complication of deep-vein sclerosis), and in some forms of vasculitis. It may also be of some value in hereditary angioneurotic oedema and in the relief of itching due to biliary obstruction. Also used in some aplastic anaemias. *Dose:* 2.5–10mg daily. Some androgenic side-effects may occur, but are usually mild and reversible on stopping treatment.

starch Carbohydrate granules obtained from maize, rice, wheat or potato. Widely used as absorbent dusting powder.

sterculia A natural gum that swells in water to a gelatinous mass. It is used as a bulk laxative as it increases faecal volume and promotes peristalsis. It is also used in diverticulitis and irritable bowel syndrome, and as an appetite suppressant. *Dose:* 5–10g daily.

stilboestrol A synthetic oestrogen with the actions and uses of oestradiol. *Dose:* 0.1–0.5mg daily for menopausal symptoms, but it is now prescribed less frequently. Dose in breast cancer, 10–20mg daily; in prostatic carcinoma, 3mg daily or more, although fosfestrol is often preferred. Side-effects include nausea, fluid retention, thrombosis, impotence and gynaecomastia.

streptokinase An enzyme preparation obtained from cultures of haemolytic streptoccocci. It has fibrinolytic properties, and is of value in deep vein thrombosis, pulmonary embolism and other conditions requiring fibrinolytic therapy. *Dose:* by intravenous infusion, 250 000 units or more initially, followed by maintenance doses of 100 000 units hrly for not less than 72 hrs. Side-effects are fever, rash, haemorrhage and allergic reactions.

streptokinase-streptodornase A mixture of enzymes obtained from cultures of haemolytic streptococci. It brings about the dissolution of blood clots and the liquefaction of purulent exudates, and it is used as a solution to clean foul wounds, pressure sores and ulcers.

streptomycin The first of the aminoglycoside antibiotics, but now used mainly as a second-choice drug in the treatment of tuberculosis. *Dose:* 1g daily i.m. usually in association with isoniazid. Its use requires care, as it is both ototoxic and nephrotoxic, especially in full doses, and in renal impairment. Measurement of the plasma concentration of streptomycin is advisable during treatment. Cutaneous sensitization has followed contact of the drug with the skin.

strychnine The alkaloid of nux vomica. It has a very bitter taste and it is used occasionally as a gastric tonic, but has no other therapeutic value. *Dose:* as Tincture of Nux Vomica, 0.6–2ml.

sucralfate An aluminium sucrose sulphate used in the treatment of peptic ulcer. It is not an antacid, but forms a barrier over the ulcer that is resistant to peptic attack and so promotes healing. *Dose:* 4g daily for at least 4 weeks. See page 212.

sulconazole A synthetic antifungal agent similar in actions and uses to miconazole. Applied as a 1% cream twice daily.

sulfadoxine A long-acting sulphonamide, with the general antibacterial action of the group. It has been used in the treatment of leprosy.

Dose: 1–1.5g weekly. In association with pyrimethamine, it is used in the prophylaxis and treatment of malaria, but the use of such mixed products requires great care, as severe, sometimes fatal, side-effects have occurred.

sulfametopyrazine A very long-acting sulphonamide used mainly in chronic bronchitis and urinary tract infections. *Dose:* 2g once a week. Side-effects and toxic reactions, although mainly those of the sulphonamides generally, may be linked with the slow excretion of the drug.

sulindac A non-steroidal anti-inflammatory analgesic agent with actions, uses and side-effects similar to those of naproxen. It is of value in the pain and inflammation of rheumatoid disease and acute gout. *Dose:* 200–400mg daily. It may cause gastrointestinal disturbance and occasional bleeding. See page 214.

sulphacarbamide See sulphaurea.

sulphacetamide A sulphonamide now used only as eye-drops 5–10%.

sulphadiazine One of the more active and less toxic sulphonamides; effective against streptococci, meningococci and many other organisms. It is used mainly in the treatment of severe conditions such as meningococcal meningitis. *Dose:* 6–9g daily by deep intramuscular injection or intravenous infusion for 2 days, followed by 2g orally or more daily. Side-effects are nausea, rash and blood dyscrasias.

sulphadimethoxine A long-acting sulphonamide, now used mainly in the treatment of active trachoma. *Dose:* 1–2g initially, followed by 0.5g daily. The side-effects are those of the sulphonamides generally.

sulphadimidine One of the least toxic of the sulphonamides. It is now used mainly in urinary infections, and in the prophylaxis and treatment of meningococcal meningitis. *Dose:* 2g initially, with maintenance of 1.5–4g daily orally, or by deep intramuscular or slow intravenous injection. Side-effects include nausea, drug fever, rash and leucopenia.

sulphaguanidine A sulphonamide, formerly used for acute gastrointestinal infections, but it may mask the symptoms and delay recovery. *Dose:* 9–12g daily for 3 days.

sulphamethoxazole A sulphonamide present with trimethaprim in co-trimoxazole. Occasionally used alone in urinary infections. *Dose:* 2g initially, followed by 1g twice daily. Adequate fluid intake necessary during treatment.

sulphasalazine A sulphonamide derivative which is said to be taken up selectively by the connective tissue of the intestines. It is used in the treatment and maintenance of remission in ulcerative colitis and colonic Crohn's disease. Occasionally given in rheumatoid arthritis. *Dose:* 4–8g daily initially; maintenance, 1.5–2g daily. It is also given as a 3g enema and as 500mg suppositories. Side-effects include nausea, rash, drug fever and blood dyscrasias. See mesalazine and olsalazine.

sulphathiazole One of the early sulphonamides, and survives in a few mixed products.

sulphaurea (sulphacarbamide) A sulphonamide used only in urinary tract infections, often in association with the urinary analgesic phenazopyridine. *Dose:* 1.5g daily.

sulphinpyrazone A drug related to phenylbutazone, but with the selective action of increasing the excretion of uric acid, hence used in the treatment of chronic gout and hyperuricaemia. *Dose:* 100–200mg initially with food, increased according to the plasma uric acid levels up to 600–800mg daily, with lower maintenance doses according to need and response. Side-effects are nausea, abdominal pain and rash. Care is necessary in peptic ulcer and renal impairment, and blood counts are necessary during treatment. Salicylates antagonize the action of the drug.

sulphonamides A group of drugs that have an antibacterial action by preventing the uptake and use of folic acid. They are thus bacteriostatic and not bactericidal in action. Although effective in a wide range of infections, the use of the sulphonamides has declined, and they are now used mainly in urinary tract infections due to sulphonamide-sensitive bacteria. The members of the group differ mainly in the rate of absorption and excretion, and so in frequency of dose. Sulphadiazine and sulphadimidine can be regarded as standard sulphonamides; sulphadimethoxine is a long-acting drug; the poorly-absorbed sulphonamides formerly used in intestinal infections are calcium sulphoxalate, phthalylsulphathiazole and sulphaguanidine. The side-effects of the sulphonamides include nausea, dyspepsia, diarrhoea and allergic reactions. Bone marrow depression may occur if treatment is prolonged. The uncommon Stevens-Johnson syndrome is a very serious reaction. See co-trimoxazole.

sulphonylureas A group of orally-active drugs represented by chlorpropamide that promote the release of insulin from the beta-cells of the pancreas. They are used in mild diabetes not controlled by diet, and in the late-onset diabetes of middle age, but they are not suitable for the treatment of juvenile diabetes. The presence of some still-functioning beta-cells is essential for sulphonylurea activity. Side-effects include weight gain, rash, fever and jaundice. During illness and pregnancy, insulin treatment should replace sulphonylurea therapy. See page 187.

sulphur A greenish-yellow, insoluble substance once used as sulphur ointment for scabies. It is also present in some products of alleged value in acne. Sulphur has also been used as a laxative in doses of 1–4g.

sulpiride An antipsychotic drug with a central action on dopamine receptors. It is used in the treatment of acute and chronic schizophrenia, as in low doses it increases awareness in apathetic and withdrawn patients, and in larger doses controls the active forms of the illness. *Dose:* 400–800mg daily: in severe conditions up to 2.4g daily. The side-effects are similar to those of chlorpromazine. See page 216.

sultamicin A pro-drug that, after absorption, yields ampicillin and the enzyme inhibitor sulbactam. The mixture increases the activity of the antibiotic. See co-amoxiclav.

suramin A drug used in the early treatment of trypanosomiasis, but it is of no value in the later stages of the disease as it does not enter the cerebrospinal fluid. *Dose:* 1g intravenously weekly for 5 weeks, after a tolerance test dose of 200mg. Side-effects are gastro-intestinal disturbances, dermatitis, hyperaesthesia and albuminuria.

suxamethonium A short-acting, depolarizing muscle relaxant, with an action lasting 3–5 min. A preliminary injection of thiopentone should first be given, as the initial effect of suxamethonium is a painful muscle contraction before the relaxant action supervenes. *Dose:* 20–100mg intravenously during surgery, with further doses according to need. Suxamethonium may also be given as a 0.1% solution by i.v. infusion. Exceptionally, the muscle relaxant action of the drug may be prolonged with marked apnoea. Unlike non-depolarizing muscle relaxants, the action of suxamethonium cannot be reversed. Severe hepatic disease is a contra-indication.

sumatriptan A serotonin-like agent with a selective vasoconstrictor action on cranial vessels. It is used in the treatment (not prophylaxis) of migraine and cluster headache, as it relieves the associated cranial vasodilatation. *Dose:* 6mg by subcutaneous injection from an auto-injector, as soon as possible after onset of an attack. Not more than two doses in 24 hours. Side-effects are mild and include injection site pain, tingling, drowsiness and weakness. Not to be used with ergotamine. (See page 204.)

sympathomimetics Drugs that have an action similar to adrenaline, and act on both alpha- and beta-adrenoceptors. More selective compounds, such as salbutamol, act on the beta$_2$-adrenoceptors in the lungs and have an increased bronchodilator action. They also relax uterine muscle, and are used to prevent premature labour.

T

talampicillin A pro-drug form of ampicillin. After absorption, it is metabolized to release ampicillin, and high plasma levels are obtained with doses of 750mg–1.5g daily. The side-effects are those of ampicillin, but talampicillin is less likely to cause diarrhoea.

talc A form of magnesium silicate, widely used as a skin dusting powder. It has also been used as a lubricant for surgeons' gloves, but it may cause a talc granuloma if any reaches the tissues during operation, and glove powders prepared from starch are preferred.

tamoxifen An oestrogen-antagonist used mainly in breast cancer, particularly when metastases are present. *Dose:* 20–40mg daily. It is usually well tolerated, but side-effects include hot flushes, dizziness, rash, hypercalcaemia and an increase in tumour pain. Unlike other oestrogen-antagonists, tamoxifen has no androgenic properties. It has also been used in some forms of anovulatory sterility.

tannic acid An astringent obtained from oak galls. Suppositories of tannic acid are used in the astringent treatment of haemorrhoids, and the acid has also been used as an oral antidote in the emergency treatment of acute alkaloid poisoning.

teicoplanin An antibiotic that acts by interfering with bacterial cell wall development. It has a wide range of activity, but is used mainly in the treatment of severe staphylococcal infections that fail to respond to other antibiotics. *Dose:* 400mg initially by intravenous injection, followed by 200mg as a single daily dose, which may be given by intramuscular injection. Double doses in severe infections. Side-effects include gastro-intestinal disturbances, dizziness, fever and rash.

temazepam A mild hypnotic of the nitrazepam type, but with a shorter duration of action. It is useful in the insomnia of the elderly, and is also of value as a pre-operative anxiolytic agent. *Dose:* 10–30mg. Daytime drowsiness is less common than with related drugs.

temofloxacin An antibacterial of the enoxacin type, with similar actions, uses and side-effects. *Dose:* 300–600mg twice a day for 14 days.

tenoxicam A non-steroidal anti-inflammatory drug (NSAID) with the actions, uses and side-effects of that group. *Dose:* 20mg as a single daily dose.

terazocin An alpha-receptor antagonist used in hypertension. It produces a peripheral vasodilatation by a blockade of post-synaptic alpha-receptors. *Dose:* 1mg *at night* initially, slowly increased up to 10mg as a single daily dose. Small initial doses are necessary to avoid episodes of syncope during early treatment. Reduced doses are indicated when terazocin is given with thiazide diuretics or other antihypertensive agents. Side-effects are dizziness, drowsiness and peripheral oedema. See prazocin.

terbinafine An antifungal agent that acts by interfering with the synthesis of ergosterol, an essential constituent of fungal cell membranes. It is used in fungal infections of the skin and nails, but it is not effective in pityriasis (*Tinea versicolor*). *Dose:* 250mg daily for 2–6 weeks; half doses in severe liver or renal impairment. Side-effects are rash, loss of appetite and gastro-intestinal disturbances.

terbutaline A selective beta-adrenoceptor stimulant and bronchodilator, with the actions, uses and side-effects of salbutamol. *Dose:* 10–15mg orally daily; by aerosol inhalation; 250–500μg by subcutaneous, intramuscular or intravenous injection.

terfenadine An antihistamine with reduced sedative and other side-effects on the central nervous system. It is effective in hayfever, allergic skin conditions and other allergic states, but it is of no value in non-allergic pruritus. *Dose:* 120mg daily.

terlipressin A synthetic form of vasopressin, used to control bleeding from oesophageal varices. *Dose:* 1–2mg intravenously, repeated if required 4–6 hrly.

terolidine An anticholinergic

agent with a relaxant effect on the detrusor muscle. It is used in the control of urinary frequency and neurogenic bladder in adults. *Dose:* 25–50mg daily. Side-effects are dryness of the mouth and visual disturbances.

testosterone The androgenic hormone of the testes, which controls the development of the male sex characteristics. It is used mainly in the treatment of hypogonadism by the i.m. injection of depot preparations of long-acting testosterone derivatives. Subcutaneous implantation of testosterone pellets (200–600mg) has been used in the treatment of metastatic breast cancer. Side-effects are weight gain, virilism and hypercalcaemia.

tetanus vaccine A preparation of tetanus toxin that has been modified by treatment with formaldehyde. It is used for active immunization against tetanus. *Dose:* 0.5ml by deep s.c. or i.m. bed vaccine containing a mineral carrier such as aluminium sulphate is often preferred.

tetrabenazine A drug of the haloperidol type, but used mainly in the treatment of Huntington's chorea and similar disorders of movement. *Dose:* 75–200mg daily. It may cause drowsiness and extrapyramidal side-effects.

tetracosactrin A synthetic form of corticotrophin, with similar actions and uses. Of value in patients allergic or unresponsive to natural corticotrophin. *Dose:* up to 2mg daily i.m. injection. It is also given as a single injection of 250μg as a test of adrenal cortex function, as after such an injection, the level of cortisol in the plasma should rise within an hour.

tetracycline A wide-range antibiotic very similar both chemically and pharmacologically to chlortetracycline, oxytetracycline, clomocycline, and related compounds referred to generically as the tetracyclines. They all have the same type of action against both Gram-positive and Gram-negative organisms, but exhibit certain differences in solubility, absorption and excretion. These differences are reflected in the different doses, as tetracycline is given in doses of 250mg four times a day, whereas with doxycycline a single daily dose of 100mg may be adequate. Long treatment with a tetracycline may lead to gastrointestinal disturbance owing to changes in the normal bacterial population of the intestinal tract. The use of the tetracyclines has declined with the emergence of bacterial resistance. They also have the disadvantage of being taken up and staining growing teeth and bone, and so should not be given to children or used during pregnancy. The absorption of the tetracyclines is reduced by antacids, calcium, iron and milk. See Table 30, page 267.

theophylline A bronchodilator with the actions and uses of aminophylline. It is used mainly in the less severe forms of asthma and respiratory disease. *Dose:* 180mg–1g daily. Side-effects include gastro-intestinal disturbances and tachycardia, but such reactions are less frequent when long-acting preparations of theophylline are used. Such preparations are also useful in the control of nocturnal asthma.

thiabendazole An anthelmintic effective against a wide range of intestinal parasites. Also useful in creeping eruption. *Dose:* 50mg/kg daily, up to a maximum of 3g daily for 2–3 days. Side-effects are nausea, diarrhoea, rash, yellow vision and jaundice.

thiamine Also known as aneurine and vitamin B_1. It is essential for carbohydrate metabolism, but is used clinically mainly in cases of deficiency, as in beri-beri, or when the diet is restricted. Also of value in the neuritis of pregnancy and alcoholism. *Dose:* 2–5mg daily; therapeutic, 25–100mg daily, in severe deficiency 200–300mg daily.

thiazides See diuretics.

thiethylperazine An anti-emetic which although related to chlorpromazine, has no tranquillizing properties. It acts centrally by inhibiting the stimulation of the chemoreceptor trigger zone, and is of value in nausea, vertigo and labyrinthine disorders, and in controlling the vomiting induced by cytotoxic therapy. *Dose:* 20–30mg daily, or 6.5mg by i.m. injection or as a suppository. Side-effects include drowsiness, hypotension and dryness of the mouth. In young women and debilitated patients it may cause extra-pyramidal symptoms.

thioguanine A cytotoxic agent similar in action and uses to mercaptopurine, and used to induce and maintain remission in acute myeloblastic and other leukaemias. *Dose:* 2mg/kg daily. Side-effects are bone marrow depression, nausea and jaundice.

thiopentone A widely used, short-acting intravenous anaesthetic. *Dose:* 100–150mg initially, repeated at intervals of 20–30 seconds as required. Solutions should be freshly prepared, and great care must be taken to avoid extravasation, as the solution is very alkaline and may cause tissue necrosis. Intra-arterial injection is also dangerous.

thioridazine A tranquillizing

drug related to chlorpromazine, and used in similar doses for the treatment of schizophrenia and other psychiatric conditions. Unlike most related drugs, it has no anti-emetic properties. *Dose:* 30–600mg daily.

thiotepa A cytotoxic drug similar in action to mustine, but not irritant. Used in a variety of cancerous conditions. *Dose:* by intravenous injection, 15–30mg, repeated according to the response. Larger doses have been injected directly into tumours. It is sometimes given by intrathecal injection in doses up to 10mg. Thiotepa is also given by intra-cavity instillation in doses of 10–30mg in the treatment of malignant effusions, and up to 90mg are used for bladder instillation. Side-effects are bone marrow depression, nausea and alopecia.

thymoxamine A peripheral vasodilator that is useful in vasospasm and other peripheral ischaemic conditions. *Dose:* 160mg daily. It is sometimes used as eye-drops (0.5%) to reverse the mydriatic action of phenylephrine. Side-effects such as headache and facial flushing are usually mild and transient.

thyroxine The active constituent of thyroid, but now prepared synthetically. Thyroxine is a powerful metabolic stimulant, specific in neonatal hypothyroidism (cretinism) and myxoedema. *Dose:* in the former, early diagnosis and treatment are essential to ensure normal development, and therapy can be commenced with an initial dose of 10μg/kg. In thyroid deficiency states generally, 100μg daily may be given initially, with subsequent maintenance doses of up to 200μg daily. Overdose, or too-rapid treatment may cause palpitations, flushing and diarrhoea.

tiaprofenic acid A non-steroidal analgesic and anti-inflammatory agent with the actions, uses and side-effects of related NSAIDs such as naproxen. *Dose:* 600–800mg daily. Mild oedema may occur with extended treatment. Peptic ulcer and asthma are contra-indications.

tibolone A new compound described as an gonadomimetic steroid. It is used to control the vasomotor symptoms of the menopause, including those surgically induced as well as those occurring naturally. *Dose:* 2.5mg daily for some months. Side-effects are headache, dizziness and vaginal bleeding. Treatment should be withdrawn if any thromboembolic symptoms or jaundice appears.

ticarcillin An antibiotic with the actions and uses of carbenicillin, but with an increased activity against *Pseudomonas aeruginosa.* In pseudomonal septicaemia, combined treatment with an aminoglycoside antibiotic such as gentamicin may evoke an increased response. *Dose:* 15–20g daily by slow intravenous injection or infusion in systemic infections; 3–4g daily by intramuscular injection in urinary infections. It is sometimes given together with clavulanic acid. Side-effects are those of the penicillins generally.

timolol A beta-adrenergic blocking agent of the propranolol type, used in the control of angina and hypertension. *Dose:* 10–60mg daily. In the prophylactic treatment of migraine, 10–20mg daily. Care is necessary in bradycardia, cardiac insufficiency and bronchial disease. It is also of value as eye-drops (0.25%–0.5%) in simple chronic glaucoma, as it reduces intra-ocular pressure by reducing the formation of the aqueous humour.

tinidazole A drug similar to metronidazole, and used mainly in the prophylaxis and treatment of anaerobic infections. *Dose:* 2g initially, followed by 1g daily for 5 days. A single oral dose of 2g is given 12 hrs before abdominal surgery, and a similar single dose is given in giardiasis. Side-effects are nausea, vomiting and diarrhoea. Hypersensitivity reactions may occur, but are less common.

tioconazole An antifungal agent used in tinea infections of the nails by the extended application of a 28% solution. Treatment for 6 months or more may be necessary.

titanium dioxide A metallic oxide, similar to zinc oxide, with mild astringent properties. It is present in some sunburn protection preparations.

tobramycin An aminoglycoside antibiotic with the actions, uses and side-effects of gentamicin, but considered to be more active against *Pseudomonas aeruginosa.* *Dose:* 3–5mg/kg daily by intramuscular injection or intravenous infusion. It may be given together with a penicillin or metronidazole in serious mixed infections. Care is necessary to avoid the ototoxic and nephrotoxic effects of aminoglycosides.

tocainide An anti-arrhythmic agent similar in action to lignocaine. It is a powerful drug, and may cause severe blood disturbances, and its use is largely restricted to the control of life-threatening arrhythmias not responding to other drugs. *Dose:* 500–750mg by slow i.v. injection or infusion, followed by 600–800mg orally and maintenance doses of 1.2g daily. Blood counts during treatment are essential. Side-effects include bradycardia, hypotension, rash, tremor and aplastic anaemia.

tocopherol A synthetic form of vitamin E.

tolazamide An oral hypoglycaemic agent related to tolbutamide, with similar actions, uses and side-effects. *Dose:* 100–250mg daily, increased if necessary up to a maximum dose of 1g daily. See Table 12 on page 190.

tolbutamide A sulphonylurea used like chlorpropamide in the treatment of maturity-onset diabetes, but it has a shorter action, and twice-daily doses are usually necessary. It is effective only when some insulin-secreting cells of the pancreas are still functioning, and a return to insulin therapy may be necessary during illness and infection. Tolbutamide is not suitable for the treatment of juvenile or severe diabetes. *Dose:* 0.5–2g daily. Side-effects include hypoglycaemia, rash, jaundice and blood dyscrasias, but are uncommon with low doses. See Table 12 on page 190.

tolbuterol A beta$_2$ adrenergic agonist used in the prophylaxis and treatment of bronchospasm in asthma and related conditions. *Dose:* 4–6mg daily. Side-effects are headache, tremor, tachycardia and central stimulation. It may precipitate angina.

tolmetin An anti-inflammatory analgesic agent used in rheumatoid and musculoskeletal conditions. As with related NSAIDs it may cause gastrointestinal disturbances in some patients, and should be taken after food. Hypersensitivity reactions may occur occasionally. *Dose:* 0.6–1.8g daily.

tolnaftate A synthetic antifungal agent used topically as a 1% cream in tinea and other fungal infections of the skin. Hypersensitivity reactions may occur, but are uncommon.

tranquillizers These drugs were once separated into the major tranquillizers, represented by chlorpromazine, and the minor tranquillizers exemplified by diazepam, but are now often referred to as antipsychotic drugs and anxiolytics respectively. The antipsychotics are used mainly in the control of disturbed patients, and in schizophrenia, although they have some anti-anxiety properties, and long-term treatment is often necessary. The anxiolytic drugs are intended mainly for the short-term treatment of acute anxiety states, as extended use may cause dependence.

tranexamic acid An antifibrinolytic agent used to check haemorrhage after prostatectomy, in surgery generally and in the control of menorrhagia. *Dose:* 2–6g daily; 3g daily by slow intravenous injection. Side-effects are nausea, diarrhoea and dizziness. Myalgia may occur, and although uncommon, indicates withdrawal of the drug.

Transiderm-Nitro A medicated patch containing glyceryl trinitrate designed to have an action over 24 hrs in the prophylaxis of angina.

tranylcypromine A monoamine oxidase inhibitor, of use in severe depression not responding to other drugs. *Dose:* 20mg daily initially, increased to 30mg daily or more according to need. The use of tranylcypromine requires care, as the drug has a stimulant action that may complicate therapy, and phenelzine may be preferred. Side-effects are dizziness, dry mouth and insomnia. Liver damage may also occur, and a hypertensive crisis requires withdrawal of the drug. Hyperthyroidism is a contra-indication.

trazodone An antidepressant chemically distinct from other drugs with a similar action, and with reduced anticholinergic and cardiovascular side-effects. It is indicated mainly in depression associated with anxiety when a sedative action is also required. *Dose:* 150–300mg daily. The side-effects are those of the tricyclic antidepressants such as amitriptyline.

treosulfan A cytotoxic agent related to busulphan, but used mainly in ovarian cancer. *Dose:* 1–2g daily for 28 days, repeated after a 4-week rest period; 5–15g by intravenous injection at intervals of 1–3 weeks. In all cases the dose is adjusted according to the degree of bone marrow depression that occurs. Other side-effects are those of cytotoxic drugs generally. Extravasation causes pain and local tissue damage.

tretinoin A vitamin A derivative used as lotion or gel (0.025%) in the treatment of acne. It may cause some redness of the skin.

triamcinolone A glucocorticosteroid with the actions, uses and side-effects of hydrocortisone, but differing by promoting sodium excretion, and so is of no value in adrenal cortex deficiency states. It is used in a wide range of inflammatory, allergic and respiratory states, and in inflammatory skin conditions. *Dose:* 8–24mg daily. It is also given as triamcinolone acetonide in doses of 40mg by deep intramuscular injection for a depot action. The acetonide is also given by intra-articular injection in doses of 2.5–40mg in local inflammation of the joints, and by intra-lesional injection in dose of 2–3mg at any one site for the treatment of skin lesions. Triamcinolone acetonide is also used as a 1% cream or ointment in severe inflammatory skin conditions. The side-effects are those of the corticosteroids (see hydrocortisone), but triamcinolone may also cause myopathy with high dose treatment.

triamterene A potassium-sparing diuretic, used mainly in association with more powerful drugs. It is indicated in oedematous conditions generally, and as it causes some retention of potassium, its use avoids the need for supplementary potassium therapy. *Dose:* 150–250mg daily, with lower doses for the elderly, and when given in association with other diuretics. Rash and gastrointestinal disturbances are side-effects.

triazolam An hypnotic of the nitrazepam type, but effective in much smaller doses. It has been used for the short-term treatment of insomnia in elderly patients, as an extended response is unlikely. It has caused psychological disturbances in some patients, and it has recently been withdrawn. Its safety is under review. *Dose:* 125–250μg.

tribavarin An inhibitor of viral replication used in severe viral bronchiolitis in infants. It is given by aerosol inhalation of a solution (20mg/ml) for 12–18 hrs daily for 3–7 days, together with supportive therapy.

trichloroacetic acid Deliquescent crystals, used as a powerful caustic for warts.

trichloroethylene A liquid sometimes used by inhalation to supplement nitrous oxide-oxygen anaesthesia. It should not be used in closed circuit apparatus, as toxic breakdown products may be formed. It has some analgesic properties, and small doses by inhalation have been used in trigeminal neuralgia. Trichlorethylene is widely used in industry and dry-cleaning, and prolonged exposure may lead to chronic poisoning with both cardio-toxic and neurotoxic effects.

triclofos A derivative of chloral, with the sedative properties of the parent drug, but is less irritant to the gastric mucosa. *Dose:* 1–2g.

triclosan A chlorinated phenolic antiseptic, used mainly in surgical scrubs and similar preparations.

Tridil Glyceryl trinitrate, prepared for intravenous infusion in the treatment of refractory angina, and in myocardial ischaemia. The solution, containing 50mg/10mL must be diluted with sterile water or saline before use to a concentration of 400μg/ml, or less. It is then given by intravenous infusion in carefully controlled doses of 10–200μg/min according to need and response.

trientine A copper-chelating agent used in Wilson's disease, but only for patients unable to tolerate penicillamine. *Dose:* 1.2–2.4g daily. It is not an alternative to penicillamine in other conditions. The main side-effect is nausea.

trifluoperazine A powerful tranquillizing drug of the chlorpromazine type. It is used mainly in schizophrenia and similar psychoses, and in severe anxiety. *Dose:* 10–20mg or more daily according to need. In severe anxiety, 2–6mg daily. In acute conditions, 1–3mg daily by deep intramuscular injection. As an anti-emetic, it is given in doses of 2–4mg or 1–3mg by injection. The side-effects are similar to those of chlorpromazine, including extrapyramidal symptoms, but the anticholinergic and sedative side-effects are less severe.

trifluperidol A powerful tranquillizer of the haloperidol type, with similar actions, uses and side-effects, including extrapyramidal symptoms. It is used mainly in schizophrenia and mania. *Dose:* 1–6mg daily according to need and response.

tri-iodothyronine See liothyronine.

trilostane An inhibitor of enzyme systems concerned with production of mineralo- and glucocorticosteroids by the adrenal cortex, and so resembles metyrapone to some extent. It is used to control adrenal cortex hyperfunction and the excessive production of aldosterone. *Dose:* 240mg daily initially, adjusted up to a maximum of 480mg daily, according to the plasma corticosteroid levels. Care is necessary in liver and kidney dysfunction.

trimeprazine A sedative antihistamine used in the treatment of pruritus and allergic itching conditions, and for premedication. *Dose:* 30–100mg daily; pre-medication dose: 3mg/kg.

trimetaphan A short-acting ganglionic-blocking agent. It is used to produce a controllable reduction in blood pressure during neuro- and vascular surgery when a relatively bloodless field is necessary. *Dose:* by intravenous infusion, 3–4mg/minute initially, with subsequent doses carefully adjusted to the response. Side-effects are tachycardia and respiratory depression. Frequent determination of blood pressure during use is essential.

trimethoprim An antibacterial agent similar in action to the sulphonamides. It is used in the prophylaxis and treatment of urinary tract and respiratory infections due to sensitive bacteria. Dose in chronic infections: 200–400mg daily: prophylactic dose 100mg daily. In severe infections, 150–250mg twice daily by slow intravenous injection. Side-effects are nausea, vomiting, rash and pruritus, and possible bone marrow depression. See co-trimoxazole.

trimipramine A sedative antidepressant with the action and side-effects of amitriptyline. It is valuable in depression complicated by anxiety. *Dose:* 75–300mg daily.

triple vaccine Diphtheria, tetanus and pertussis vaccine for the primary immunization of children. *Dose:* 0.5ml by i.m. or deep s.c. injection.

triprolidine An antihistamine used for the relief of allergic conditions generally. *Dose:* 7.5–15mg daily. Side-effects are dryness of the mouth, drowsiness and blurred vision.

trisodium edetate A chelating or binding agent that is sometimes used in hypercalcaemia. The calcium complex so formed is excreted in the urine. Dose by slow intravenous infusion up to 70mg/kg daily according to need and response, as shown by plasma calcium measurement. It is also used as a 0.4% solution for opththalmic use in lime burns of the eyes. Side-effects after injection are nausea, diarrhoea and cramp. Contra-indicated in renal impairment.

tropicamide A short-acting mydriatic agent similar to homatropine. Used as 0.5% and 1% solution.

tryparsamide Used in late trypanosomiasis when the CNS is involved. *Dose:* 1–3g by injection weekly, up to a maximum of 24g. May damage optic nerves.

tuberculin A product obtained from cultures of *Mycobacterium tuberculosis.* It is used in the diagnosis of tuberculosis, often as tuberculin PPD (purified protein derivative), by the intradermal injection of a 1:1000 solution (the Mantoux test). A positive reaction is the development of a papule at the injection site, and is considered to be indicative of an infection by the tubercle bacillus, although the infection may be inactive. See BCG vaccine.

tubocurarine The non-depolarizing muscle relaxant obtained from curare (once used as an arrow poison). It is widely used in general anaesthesia to increase muscle relaxation during major surgery, and has a medium-to-long duration of action, but assisted respiration is usually required. *Dose:* 15–25mg initially i.v. with supplementary doses at intervals of about 20 min, up to a total of 45mg if required. The response is increased by some inhalation anaesthetics, and by gentamicin-like antibiotics. The action can be reversed by neostigmine. Side-effects are a transient fall in blood pressure and a rash on the neck and chest, which is associated with some release of histamine. Reduced doses should be given in renal impairment.

tyrothricin A minor antibiotic used as lozenges for mouth infections.

U

undecenoic acid An organic acid with useful antimycotic properties. It is used mainly as powder or ointment (5%), often with zinc undecenoate in the treatment of athlete's foot and associated conditions.

urea An osmotic diuretic formerly used by injection to reduce cerebral oedema. Mannitol is now preferred. *Dose:* 40–80g as a 30% solution in 5% glucose by intravenous infusion. It has also been used orally as a diuretic in doses of 5–15g. Applied locally as a 10% solution, it promotes granulation and reduces odour from foul ulcers.

urofollitrophin A preparation of human follicle-stimulating hormone (FSH) used with menotrophin for the induction of ovulation. Dose and duration of treatment requires careful control to avoid over-stimulation.

urokinase A plasmin activator obtained from human urine. It is used mainly in the thrombolysis of blocked intravenous shunts, and in the lysis of blood clots in the eye. *Dose:* 5000–37,500 units, instilled into the shunt; similar doses are injected into the anterior chamber of the eye for the resolution of blood clots.

ursodeoxycholic acid The acid appears to be a solvent of cholesterol, and is given orally to promote the dissolution of cholesterol-containing gallstones. *Dose:* 8–12mg/kg as a single daily dose, but prolonged treatment is required, which should be continued after the dissolution of the stones to inhibit recurrence. The dissolution of calcium-containing or radio-opaque stones is unlikely to occur.

V

vaccines Bacterial vaccines are suspensions or extracts of dead bacteria, but some antiviral vaccines are also available. They may be given by s.c. or i.m. injection, and are used mainly for prophylaxis against a particular infection. The most commonly used vaccines include typhoid, cholera, diphtheria, influenza, tetanus and polio vaccines. Protection against mumps, measles, pertussis, rubella, yellow fever and hepatitis can also be obtained. The so-called allergen vaccines, used for desensitization to various allergens such as grass pollens, are not true vaccines, but weak solutions of allergen extracts. They may precipitate allergic reactions in susceptible patients, and should be used only when emergency resuscitation measures are immediately available.

vancomycin An antibiotic used in overwhelming staphylococcal infections resistant to other antibiotics. It is also used in the control of bacterial endocarditis. *Dose:* 2g daily by i.v. infusion. It is also used in staphylococcal enteritis and pseudomembranous colitis. *Dose:* 0.5g orally daily. Care is necessary in renal impairment, and blood concentrations of the drug should be monitored. Side-effects after injection include nausea, chills, fever and urticaria. Vancomycin is also ototoxic, and tinnitus is an indication that the drug should be withdrawn. Too rapid an injection may cause a generalized rash. Extravasation may cause necrosis and thrombophlebitis at the injection site. See teicoplanin.

vasoconstrictors Drugs such as noradrenaline that constrict the peripheral vessels, and so cause a temporary rise in blood pressure. They are useful in hypotensive conditions when the blood volume is still adequate, and in controlling the fall in blood pressure that occurs in spinal and general anaesthesia. They were widely used in the treatment of shock, but the rise in blood pressure that they produce is linked with a fall in pressure in vital organs such as the kidneys, and in shock reliance is now largely based on drugs such as isoprenaline and dopamine, together with plasma expanders such as dextran.

vasodilators Traditional vasodilators used in the prophylaxis and treatment of angina include glyceryl trinitrate and other nitrates. They have a general effect on the venous system but newer and more selectively acting antihypertensive drugs are the beta-adrenoreceptor blocking agents represented by propranolol, and the calcium-channel blocking agents such as nifedipine. Other vasodilators include drugs such as the alpha-adrenoceptor blocking agents (indoramin, prazosin) and the ACE inhibitors (captopril). Cerebral vasodilators are represented by isoxsuprine. Peripheral vasodilators include cinnarizine and thymoxamine. Many other antihypertensive drugs also have a vasodilator action.

vasopressin A preparation of the blood pressure-raising and antidiuretic factors of the pituitary gland. It has been used in doses of 5–20 units twice daily by s.c. or i.m. injection in diabetes insipidus, but has been largely superseded by demopressin.

vecuronium A non-depolarizing muscle relaxant of the tubocurarine type. It has a medium duration of action, with the advantage of not causing histamine release. *Dose:* 80–100μg/kg initially, with supplementary doses of 30–50μg/kg as required.

verapamil A calcium-channel blocking agent that reduces the movement of calcium ions in cardiac tissues. It reduces the oxygen demand as well as reducing the contractility of the myocardium, and it is used in angina, arrhythmias and hypertension. *Dose:* 120–480mg daily according to the condition and degree of response. In severe arrhythmias, 5–10mg i.v. under ECG control. Contra-indicated in bradycardia, heart failure and heart block. Side-effects include nausea, hypotension and heart block. It should be used with caution in a patient already receiving a beta-adrenoceptor blocking agent.

vidarabine An antiviral agent used mainly in the early treatment of serious herpes virus infections in immunocompromised patients. *Dose:* in chicken-pox and herpes zoster infections, 10mg/kg daily by IV infusion for at least 5 days, with smaller doses in cases of renal impairment. It depresses bone marrow function, and blood counts are necessary during treatment. Side-effects are nausea, diarrhoea and confusion. Vidarabine is also used as a 3% eye ointment for herpes simplex keratoconjunctivitis and dendritic corneal ulcer.

vigabatrin A new anti-epileptic drug. GABA (a form of aminobutyric acid) is an inhibitor of neurotransmission, and epileptic seizures may be linked with a GABA deficiency. Vigabatrin has an inhibitory action on the GABA-metabolizing enzyme, and so indirectly permits a rise in the brain level of

GABA. It is used in the treatment of epilepsy not responding to other anticonvulsants. *Dose:* 2g daily initially, with adjustments up to 4g daily. Side-effects are numerous, and include drowsiness, fatigue, dizziness and weight gain. Sudden withdrawal is inadvisable. See page 192.

viloxazine An antidepressant with the general action, uses and side-effects of amitriptyline, but with a reduced sedative activity. It is given in depression associated with apathy, and in the depression of epilepsy. *Dose:* 150–400mg daily. It may increase the action of phenytoin and antihypertensive agents.

vinblastine An alkaloid of periwinkle that has cytotoxic properties. It is used in the control of acute leukaemias, lymphomas and other malignant conditions, and in mycosis fungoides. *Dose:* 100μg/kg weekly i.v. increased by 50μg/kg weekly up to 500μg/kg weekly according to response. Side-effects include myelosuppression, neurotoxicity and abdominal disturbances. The drug should be handled with care as it is a tissue irritant.

vincristine A vinca alkaloid with the action and uses of vinblastine, but much less likely to cause myelodepression. It is used mainly in the treatment of acute leukaemias in children, Hodgkin's disease and other malignant lymphomas. *Dose:* 50μg/kg by i.v. injection weekly initially, adjusted according to need up to a maximum of 150μg/kg weekly. Neuromuscular side-effects may limit the dose. Other side-effects are abdominal disturbance and alopecia. The injection of the drug requires care as it is a tissue irritant.

vindesine A vinca alkaloid with an action similar to that of vincristine. It is used mainly in acute lymphoblastic leukaemia in children, and in other malignant conditions not responding to treatment. *Dose:* 3mg/m^2 weekly by i.m. injection, subsequently increased up to 5mg/m^2 according to response. The side-effects are similar to those of other vinca alkaloids, but granulocytopenia may be a dose-limiting factor. Extravasation should be avoided, as it may cause considerable local irritation.

vitamin A One of the vitamins obtained from fish-liver oils. A deficiency in the diet causes night-blindness, skin changes and a decrease resistance to infection. *Dose:* 2500–25 000 units daily.

vitamin B A group of water-soluble vitamins obtained from yeast or rice polishings. The constituents include thiamine, riboflavine, nicotinic acid, pyridoxine, and small amounts of other factors.

vitamin B_6 Pyridoxine.

vitamin B_{12} Cyanocobalamin.

vitamin C Ascorbic acid.

vitamin D The vitamin essential for the absorption of calcium and phosphorus and subsequent bone formation. Several forms of the vitamin are known, but it is used chiefly as calciferol. Vitamin D is activated in the liver and kidneys to more powerful derivatives such as calcitriol and alfacalcidol.

vitamin D_2 Calciferol.

vitamin E The vitamin in the germ of wheat, rice and other grains. Deficiency states are uncommon, but may occur in cystic fibrosis and other conditions where fat absorption is impaired. It has been used empirically in many other conditions, but its therapeutic value is questionable. *Dose:* 5–15mg daily. Now largely replaced by the synthetic form tocopherol.

vitamin K The vitamin concerned with the formation of prothrombin, and so with blood coagulation. Given as menadiol in haemorrhagic disorders, vitamin K_1 or phytomenadione has a similar but more rapid and sustained action. Of no value when the prothrombin level of the blood is adequate.

W

warfarin A synthetic anticoagulant similar to phenindione, but with reduced side-effects and it is now the preferred drug. It is used mainly in deep-vein thrombosis and transient brain ischaemia, in doses based on the prothrombin time as reported by the laboratory in terms of the International Normalized Ratio (INR). *Dose:* Pending INR report, 10mg daily initially for up to 3 days. Haemorrhage is the main side-effect, and may require the use of phytomenadione to control the excessive response.

Whitfield's ointment Benzoic acid 6%, salicylic acid 3%. Has keratolytic and fungicidal properties, and is used mainly for ringworm.

wool alcohols A water-in-oil emulsifying agent obtained from wool fat. It is used in many water-containing ointments, such as ointment of wool alcohols and hydrous ointment.

wool fat A pale yellow, waxy substance, also known as lanolin, obtained from sheeps' wool. It consists mainly of cholesterol-derivatives, and is a constituent of various water-in-oil emulsifying and emollient ointment bases. It may cause skin sensitization in some susceptible patients.

X

xamoterol A partial β_1 adrenoceptor agonist with a cardiac stimulant action. It is given only in mild chronic heart failure to control exercise-induced symptoms. *Dose:* 400mg daily. Side-effects are dizziness, headache and gastro-intestinal disturbances. Contra-indicated in severe heart failure, and care is necessary in asthmatic conditions.

xipamide A long-acting diuretic and antihypertensive similar to chlorthalidone. *Dose:* in hypertension, 20mg is given as a morning dose; in oedematous states, 40–80mg as a single morning dose, reduced later as necessary.

xylometazoline A sympathomimetic agent used as a nasal decongestant, and to relieve allergic conjunctivitis as drops of 0.05–0.1%. Rebound congestion may be a side-effect.

xylose A sugar used for the evaluation of intestinal absorption. Following an oral dose of 5–25g, the amount recoverable from the urine is measured, and a recovery of less than 16% of a dose is indicative of malabsorption, provided the renal function is adequate. Side-effects include nausea, abdominal discomfort and diarrhoea.

Y

yeast The fungus used in the fermentation of sugars to produce alcohol. Dried yeast has been used as dietary suplement for its vitamin B content.

Z

zidovudine An antiviral agent effective against the human immunodeficiency virus (HIV), associated with the acquired immune deficiency syndrome (AIDS). It inhibits the enzyme reverse transcriptase and, by preventing the formation of viral DNA, it inhibits viral development. *Dose:* 3.5mg/kg 4 hrly for some months. Side-effects include anaemia, neutropenia, nausea, fever and malaise. Liver-function tests are necessary during treatment. The chronic use of analgesics such as paracetamol may increase the risk of neutropenia.

zinc oxide A soft white powder widely used in dusting powders, ointments, pastes, etc., for its mild astringent and antiseptic properties. It is a constituent of Lassar's paste, Unna's paste, Calamine Lotion and similar preparations.

zinc peroxide An insoluble white powder with an antiseptic action similar to hydrogen peroxide but slower and more prolonged. Used as lotion (40%), mouthwash (25%), ointment (20%).

zinc stearate A white insoluble powder used as a mild astringent in dusting powders for eczema and associated conditions.

zinc sulphate Used as an astringent and stimulating lotion (1%) for indolent ulcers; and in conjunctivitis as eye-drops (0.25%). Doses of 220mg with meals are stated to promote healing of wounds in zinc-deficiency states.

zinc undecenoate A white insoluble powder. Constituent of dusting powders and ointments for mycotic conditions.

zuclopenthixol A powerful tranquillizing drug with actions, uses and side-effects similar to those of chlorpromazine, It is of value in schizophrenia with agitation or aggression. *Dose:* 20–30mg or more, up to 150mg daily. For depot maintenance treatment, 100–200mg or more by deep i.m. injection at intervals of 2–3 weeks, according to need and response.

Drugs and their use in some common disorders

More information about the drugs mentioned in this section is given in the main part of the book, pages 7–170.

Allergy

Allergy is a general term applied to hypersensitivity reactions. Some allergies, such as hayfever and atopic dermatitis, are well known, but the initiating factors that result in an allergic reaction may vary widely. Briefly, an allergic reaction originates by exposure to some excitant substance (an antigen), which in sensitive individuals is followed by the production of an antibody. Antigens are usually, but not necessarily, protein in origin, and some drugs can function as antigens, as can house dust. Subsequent re-exposure to the antigen may result in an antigen–antibody reaction, which is associated with the release of histamine and related substances, which then act upon various body tissues to produce the allergic attack. This may manifest in a variety of ways, such as hayfever, bronchoconstriction, rash or abdominal symptoms. In severe allergic reactions an alarming fall in blood pressure occurs, with acute asthma that requires the immediate injection of adrenaline solution. For symptomatic relief, antihistamines are widely used. They do not break the chain of antigen–antibody–histamine release, but block the access of the released histamine to the sensitive tissues. Their action is palliative and not curative, and the response to treatment is variable. They are usually effective in hayfever, urticaria and insect bites, but are of no value in allergic asthma. Some antihistamines also have a sedative action, which may be useful in urticaria, but undesirable in other conditions. This sedative side-effect is less marked with some of the newer antihistamines (see **Table 2**). In overdose they may cause convulsions in young patients. The extended local application of antihistamines should be avoided, as antihistamines may themselves cause an allergic-type dermatitis. Side-effects include dry mouth, blurred vision and occasional gastro-intestinal disturbances. Patients should be warned that drowsiness is a common side-effect that may affect car-driving ability. Attempts have been made to desensitize susceptible patients by injections of specific antigens, such as grass pollens. The method is not without risk, particularly in asthmatic patients, and should be carried out only by experts.

Table 2. Antihistamines

Approved name	Brand name	Daily dose range
acrivastine*	Semprex	24mg
astemizole*	Hismanal, Pollon-Eze	10mg
azatadine	Optimine	2–4mg
brompheniramine	Dimotane	12–32mg
cetrizine	Zirtek	10mg
chlorpheniramine	Piriton	12–16mg
clemastine	Tavegil	1–2mg
cyproheptadine	Periactin	8–32mg
dimethindene	Fenostil-Retard	5mg
diphenylpyraline	Histryl	10–20mg
loratadine	Clarityn	10mg
mebhydroline	Fabahistin	150–300mg
mezquitazine	Primalan	5–10mg
oxatomide*	Tinset	60–120mg
phenindamine*	Thephorin	100–200mg
pheniramine	Daneral SA	75–150mg
promethazine	Phenergan	20–75mg
terfenadine*	Triludan	60–120mg
trimeprazine	Vallergan	30–100mg
triprolidine	Actidil, Pro-Actidil	7.5–15mg

*Antihistamine with reduced sedative effects.

Anaemia

Anaemia is essentially a deficiency of red blood cells, and may occur as the result of a lack of certain factors such as iron, folic acid or vitamin B_{12}, or from disease in which the rate of breakdown of red cells exceeds the rate of production of new cells. Iron deficiency anaemia is the most common form, and may occur during pregnancy or as a consequence of restricted diets. Such a deficiency can be dealt with by the oral administration of a suitable iron salt, and ferrous sulphate is widely used. For patients who cannot tolerate ferrous sulphate, other salts are ferrous gluconate, fumarate and succinate. Some iron preparations for use during pregnancy also contain folic acid. Slow-release iron products are also available. In all cases of iron deficiency anaemia, oral treatment should be continued for some months to build up an adequate store of iron.

In a few cases, where oral iron therapy is not possible, iron-deficiency anaemia may be treated with an injectable iron product. Iron-dextran is a soluble complex that can be given by deep intramuscular injection, using a 'Z' injection technique to avoid staining the skin, or by slow intravenous injection. Iron-sorbitol is an alternative product but suitable only for intramuscular injection. The dose of these injectable products is based on the degree of iron deficiency, and their use requires care.

Megaloblastic anaemias are less common, and are due to a deficiency of vitamin B_{12} or of folic acid, or to a defect in the absorption or utilization of those factors, and may be secondary to treatment with cytotoxic agents such as methotrexate. Pernicious anaemia is the most common form of vitamin B_{12} deficiency, and develops insidiously as the normally ample stores of the vitamin in the liver are slowly depleted. Treatment is replacement therapy with hydroxocobalamin, which is the preferred form of vitamin B_{12}, as it is excreted more slowly than the older cyanocobalamin, and has a much longer action. Some oral preparations of vitamin B_{12} are available, but in general they are regarded as unsatisfactory for the treatment of vitamin B_{12} deficiency.

Aplastic anaemia is due to a marked reduction in the formation of red blood cell precursors, and is a disease of the bone marrow. It may occur from no known cause, or from exposure to some toxic agents, including cytotoxic drugs.

Bone marrow transplants are the only effective treatment, although some androgens such as oxymetholone and nandrolone have been used with occasional success. Sideroblastic anaemias are due to a disturbance in the normal utilization of iron, and may respond to large doses of pyridoxine. Haemolytic anaemia is characterized by an excessive breakdown of red blood cells, due to disease or toxic agents. Some of these less common anaemias may respond to corticosteroid therapy. The severe anaemia of end-stage renal disease in dialyzed patients differs from other anaemias in being due to a lack of erythropoietin, the kidney hormone that regulates red cell production by the bone marrow. It can now be treated with human erythropoietin obtained by recombinant DNA technology.

Table 3. Iron preparations

Approved names	Brand names
ferrous sulphate	Feospan, Ferrograd, Slow-Fe } sustained release products
ferrous fumarate	Feraday
	Fersamol
	Galfer
	Ferocap (sustained release product)
ferrous gluconate	Fergon
ferrous glycine sulphate	Plesmet
	Ferrocontin Continus (sustained release product)
ferrous succinate	Ferromyn
iron-polysaccharide complex	Niferex
sodium iron edetate	Sytron
iron-dextran injection	Imferon
iron-sorbitol injection	Jectofer
hydroxocobalamin	Cobalin-H, Neo-Cytamen
cyanocobalamin	Cytacon (oral), Cytamen
nandrolone	Deca-Durabolin
oxymetholone	Anapolon
pyridoxine	Benadon, Paxadon
epoetin (erythropoietin)	Eprex, Recormon

Anxiety

Anxiety states may manifest themselves in a variety of ways from a general sense of uneasiness to acute attacks. The symptoms may also vary widely, from a minor physical disturbance such as dryness of the mouth and sweating of the hands and 'butterflies in the stomach' to breathlessness, hyperventilation and lightheadedness. Emotional stress often precipitates anxiety, and drug treatment is useful when the cause of the stress is ill-defined or cannot be removed. Such treatment should always be regarded as a short-term measure, as the prolonged use of anxiolytics involves the risks of dependence and the problems of eventual withdrawal. For such short-term treatment of severe anxiety, a benzodiazepine such as diazepam is often the drug of choice, but other drugs such as buspirone are also in use. Some of the potent antipsychotic agents are also given in small doses for the relief of anxiety. The beta-blockers are occasionally useful in controlling some of the symptoms of anxiety, when the possibility of stress can be anticipated, as in public speaking or performance.

Table 4. Benzodiazepine anxiolytics

Approved name	Brand name	Daily dose range
alprazolam	Xanax	750–1500μg
bromazepam	Lexotan	3–18mg
buspirone	Buspar	15–45mg
chlordiazepoxide	Librium	30–100mg
clobazam	Frisium	20–30mg
clorazepate	Tranxene	7.5–22.5mg
diazepam	Alupram, Atensine, Solis, Valium	5–30mg
ketazolam	Anxon	15–60mg
lorazepam	Almazine, Ativan	2.5–10mg
medazepam	Nobrium	10–30mg
oxazepam	Oxanid	45–120mg

Asthma

Bronchial asthma is a spasmodic obstructive disease of the airways, and symptoms may vary from wheeziness to severe bronchoconstriction. Attacks may be precipitated by exposure to allergens, which may vary from house dust to pollen, fungal spores and animal hair. In some susceptible patients certain drugs, including aspirin, may intiate a severe asthmatic attack. Treatment is basically with drugs that have a relatively selective bronchodilatory action, and in the case of those drugs given by aerosol inhalation, patients must be given careful instruction in the use of the inhaler device if the optimum response is to be obtained. Isoprenaline was once used for its bronchodilator action in the treatment of asthma, but it has been virtually replaced by salbutamol and other more selective β_2-adrenoceptor stimulants. Adrenaline also has a powerful bronchodilator action, but it may cause cardiac arrhythmias, and it is now used mainly in acute anaphylaxis.

Salbutamol, now widely used, may be given orally, by aerosol inhalation, or, in acute conditions, by injection. Ipatropium and oxitropium are anticholinergic agents with a relatively selective bronchodilator action, and are of value in patients who cannot tolerate sympathomimatic agents of the salbutamol type. Other bronchodilators are the xanthines aminophylline and theophylline, but side-effects may limit their use. Some long-acting xanthine products have a sustained action associated with reduced side-effects, but such products are not necessarily bio-equivalent, and a change from one product to another should not be made without good cause. Corticosteroids are also of value in both the prophylaxis and treatment of asthma, and those given by inhalation are beclomethasone, betamethasone and budesonide. The recently introduced salmeterol is a derivative of salbutamol intended for use together with inhaled corticosteroid therapy in the propylactic treatment of asthma. It has a slow initial action, but twice daily treatment is claimed to give relief over 24 hrs. Other drugs for the prophylaxis of asthma are sodium cromoglycate and nedocromil, given by oral inhalation of a dry powder. Ketotifen is an antihistamine with some of the properties of sodium cromoglycate.

Table 5. Anti-asthma drugs

Approved names	Brand names	
selective β_2 stimulants		
fenoterol	Berotec	
pirbuterol	Exirel	
reproterol	Bronchodil	
rimiterol	Pulmadil	
salbutamol	Asmaven, Salbulin, Salbuvent Ventolin, Volmax	oral
	Aerolin 400, Aerolin Autohaler, Asmaven, Salbulin, Salbuvent, Ventolin	aerosol inhalation products
salmeterol	Serevent	
terbutaline	Bricanyl, Monovent	
tolbuterol	Brelomax	
other stimulants		
isoprenaline	Medihaler-Iso	
orciprenaline	Alupent	
xanthines		
aminophylline	Pecram, Phyllocontin Continus	
theophylline	Biophylline, Choledyl, Labophylline Nuelin, Lasma, Pro-Vent, Sabidal, Slo-Phyllin, Theo-Dur, Uniphylline Continus	
corticosteroids		
beclomethasone	Becotide, Becodisks, Becloforte	
betamethasone	Bextasol	
budesonide	Pulmicort	
prophylactics		
sodium cromoglycate	Intal	
ketoprofen	Zaditen	
nedocromil	Tilade	
anticholinergic agents		
ipatropium	Atrovent	
oxitropium	Oxivent	

Bell's palsy

Bell's palsy is a unilateral facial paralysis, characterized by sudden onset and pain. The cause is unknown, but the symptoms are thought to be due to local swelling and a compression of the facial nerve. Patients should be reassured that the paralysis is unrelated to stroke and spontaneous recovery usually occurs after some weeks. Corticosteroids are effective if the condition is diagnosed early, and prednisolone is given initially in doses of 40mg daily, decreasing by 10mg every 2 days for about a week. As the palsy may prevent closure of the affected eye, local treatment with artificial tears or liquid paraffin may be required.

Table 6. Drugs given for Bell's palsy

Approved names	Brand names
hypromellose (artificial tears)	Tears Naturelle Isopto Alkaline & Plain BJ6
liquid paraffin	Lacri-Lube
polyvinyl alcohol	Hypotears
prednisolone	Deltacortril, Deltastab, Precortisyl, Prednesol Sintisone

Cancer

The treatment of cancer is difficult because cancer cells are cells that have escaped from the controls that govern normal cell growth and differentiation of function. As a result, uncoordinated cell growth may develop rapidly, and cancer cells may migrate and invade other tissues. Any anti-cancer drug is therefore likely to damage normal cells, particularly actively growing cells such as those of the bone marrow, and the dose of a cytotoxic agent is often a compromise between that having the desired anti-cancer action and that causing toxicity.

The drugs used in the treatment of cancer can be divided into four main groups, which attack the cells at different points. The alkylating agents interfere with the replication and function of DNA, modify protein synthesis, and have correspondingly wide effects. The antimetabolites interfere with cell metabolism by combining with cell enzymes, or by forming abnormal proteins, or otherwise inhibiting normal development. The cytotoxic antibiotics have an action similar to that of the antimetabolites, but they also have radiomimetic properties, and combined radiotherapy may increase the risks of damage to normal cells. These antibiotics, with the exceptions of actinomycin D and bleomycin, also have undesirable cardiotoxic properties, and dosage requires careful control. Amsacrine is a synthetic cytotoxic agent with some of the properties of the antibiotic group.

The vinca alkaloids are a class apart, as they are plant substances, and act at the metaphase stage of cell division. They are used mainly in acute leukaemias and some lymphomas. Vincristine is almost free from any depressive effects on bone marrow function, vinblastine has some degree of myelosuppressive activity but is less neurotoxic. Vindesine occupies an intermediate position. Etoposide is a synthetic drug with some of the properties of the vinca alkaloids. Other and unclassified cytotoxic agents include the platinum complexes carboplatin and cisplatin, used mainly in ovarian cancer, and the enzyme cristantaspase used in acute lymphoblastic leukaemia. Some cancers are hormone dependent, and the symptoms may be controlled by suitable hormone treatment (see fosfesterol and testosterone).

Certain hormone analogues have applications in the treatment of prostatic carcinoma (see buserelin and goserelin). Some hormone antagonists have an anti-hormone action with reduced side-effects, and aminoglutethimide is a first choice drug in breast cancer, and the anti-androgen cyproterone is given in carcinoma of the prostate.

A distressing side-effect of high-dosage cytotoxic chemotherapy is severe and intractable nausea and vomiting, which may be so intense that patients may refuse further treatment. See page 208.

Table 7. Anti-cancer drugs

Approved names	Brand names
alkylating agents	
busulphan	Myleran
carmustine	BiCNU
chlorambucil	Leukeran
cyclophosphamide	Endoxana
estramustine	Estracyt
ethoglucid	Epodyl
ifosfamide	Mitoxana
lomustine	CCNU
melphalan	Alkeran
mustine	Mustine
thiotepa	Thiotepa
treosulphan	Treosulfan
antimetabolites	
cytarabine	Alexan, Cytosar
fluorouracil	Fluoro-uracil, Efudix
mercaptopurine	Puri-Nethol
methotrexate	Maxtrex
thioguanine	Lanvis
cytotoxic antibiotics	
actinomycin D	Cosmegen
bleomycin	Bleomycin
doxorubicin	Doxorubicin
epirubicin	Pharmarubicin
mitomycin	Mitomycin C
vinca alkaloids	
vinblastine	Velbe
vincristine	Oncovin
vindesine	Eldesine

Approved names	**Brand names**
other agents	
amsacrine	Amsidine
etoposide	Vepesid
carboplatin	Paraplatin
cisplatin	Cisplatin
crisantaspase	Erwinase
dacarbazine	DTIC
hydroxyurea	Hydrea
interferon	Intron-A, Roferon-A, Wellferon
mitozantrone	Novantrone
procarbazine	Natulan
razoxane	Razoxin
hormone antagonists	
aminoglutethimide	Orimeton
buserelin	Suprefact
cyproterone	Cyprostat
goserelin	Zoladex
octreotide	Sandostatin
tamoxifen	Emblon, Noltam, Nolvadex, Tamofen

Cough

Cough is an explosive expiration of air from the lungs, and is a protective mechanism to expel excessive exudate or foreign bodies from the respiratory tract, but other irritant factors may also stimulate the cough reflex. Productive cough should not be suppressed without good cause, as when the patient finds cough is exhausting or prevents sleep, but suppression may then have the undesirable effect of causing retention of sputum. On the other hand, suppression of the dry, useless or unproductive cough may have corresponding advantages. Many soothing and demulcent preparations represented by simple linctus have been used for the symptomatic relief of cough, and another traditional remedy is steam inhalation, assisted by the addition of Friar's balsam and menthol. Expectorant products such as ammonia and ipecacuanha mixture are also used, even though pharmacological proof of their efficacy may be lacking. Cough suppressants, represented by codeine, have a central depressant action on the cough centre, but effective doses may have the disadvantage of causing constipation. Extended use should be avoided because of the possible risk of habituation. The treatment of severe cough in terminal lung cancer is with more potent cough suppressants such as diamorphine or methadone.

Table 8. Cough suppressants

Approved names	Brand names
codeine linctus	Galcodine
pholcodine linctus	Galenophol, Pavocol D Pholcomed

Cystitis

Cystitis is an inflammatory disease of the lower urinary tract, more common in women, with painful urinary frequency and urgency, and often with low back pain. It is usually caused by Gram-negative bacteria, particularly *E. coli*, and first-line treatment is ample fluids. Sodium bicarbonate or potassium citrate is sometimes given to relieve the dysuria by making the urine alkaline. Uncomplicated cystitis usually responds to a wide-range antibiotic, or to trimethoprim, nitrofurantoin, co-trimoxazole, or a quinolone antibacterial agent such as nalidixic acid. Some of the quinolones are also useful for the long-term suppressive treatment of recurrent infections.

Table 9. Drugs used to treat cystitis

Approved names	Brand names
antibiotics	
ampicillin	Amifen, Penbritin, Vidopen
amoxycillin	Almodan, Amoxil
cephalosporins (see Table 29, page 267)	
quinolones	
ciprofloxacin	Ciproxin
cinoxacin	Cinobac
enoxacin	Comprecin
nalidixic acid	Mictral, Negram, Uriben
norfloxacin	Utinor
temafloxacin	Teflox
trimethoprim	Ipral, Monotrim, Syraprim, Trimogal, Trimopan
co-trimoxazole (trimethoprim with sulphamethoxazole)	Bactrim, Chemotrim, Comox, Laratrim, Septrin
nitrofurantoin	Furadantin, Macrodanton

Depression

Depression is a natural reaction to disappointment and grief, but it is normally brief and self-limiting. Excessive or prolonged depression is an illness, sometimes without apparent cause, and it appears to be linked with an imbalance in the brain of certain amine substances, including serotonin, that act as neuroregulators. Drug therapy can assist in restoring a normal balance, but prolonged treatment is usually necessary to evoke a full response. The drugs in most frequent use are the tricyclic antidepressants, so-called from their chemical structure, together with the monoamine oxidase inhibitors (MAOIs). All the tricyclic antidepressants have the same general pattern of activity, but some, such as amitriptyline are more sedative than others. Some related compounds have a similar antidepressant action, but blood counts are essential with mianserin and convulsions have been reported after maprotiline therapy. The monoamine oxidase inhibitors are phenelzine, isocarboxazid and tranylcypromine. They are now used less often, as they are potent drugs that react with many other therapeutic agents, as well as certain food such as cheese, broad beans, pickled herring, or meat/yeast extracts. Particular care is necessary with tranylcypromine. Fluvoxamine, fluoxetine, paroxetine and sertraline are newer drugs that have a more selective antidepressant action mediated by inhibiting the uptake of serotonin.

Table 10. Antidepressants

Approved name	Brand name	Daily dose range
tricyclic and similar		
[a]amitriptyline	Domical, Lentizol, Tryptizol	75–200mg
amoxapine	Asendis	100–300mg
butriptyline	Evadyne	75–150mg
clomipramine	Anafranil	30–150mg
desipramine	Pertofran	75–200mg
[a]dothiepin	Prothiaden	75–150mg
[a]doxepin	Sinequan	30–300mg
imipramine	Tofranil	75–200mg
iprindole	Prondol	45–180mg
lofepramine	Gamanil	70–210mg
[a]maprotiline	Ludiomil	25–150mg
[a,b]mianserin	Bolvidon, Norval	30–200mg
nortriptyline	Allegron, Aventyl	30–100mg
[b]protriptyline	Concordin	15–60mg
trazodone	Molipaxin	150–300mg
trimipramine	Surmontil	50–300mg
viloxazine	Vivalan	300–400mg
monoamine oxidase inhibitors		
isocarboxazid	Marplan	10–20mg
phenelzine	Nardil	15–30mg
tranylcypromine	Parnate	10–30mg
other antidepressants		
fluoxetine	Prozac	20mg
flupenthixol	Fluanxol	1–3mg
fluvoxamine	Faverin	100–200mg
paroxetine	Seroxat	20–50mg
sertraline	Lustral	50–100mg

[a]These drugs have sedative properties that are of value when depression is complicated by anxiety.
[b]Mianserin is a tetracyclic compound.

Diabetes

Diabetes mellitus is a deficiency caused by a lack of insulin, a specific hormone secreted by the islet cells of the pancreas, or by a failure of the insulin-release mechanism. As a result of that insulin deficiency, carbohydrates and fats are not fully metabolized. Glucose accumulates in the circulation and causes a diuresis, so that polyuria and thirst are troublesome complications. Insulin-dependent diabetes, which occurs mainly in children and young adults, can be controlled by injections of insulin. Soluble insulin is used for rapid treatment and in emergencies, but stabilized patients can be controlled by one of the longer-acting forms of insulin such as insulin-zinc-suspension. Insulin was once obtained from pigs or cattle, but human types of insulin are now available and used to an increasing extent. See Table 11.

In middle age, a non-insulin-dependent type of diabetes may develop. In such patients, the natural secretion of insulin still occurs, but the insulin is not released according to metabolic requirements. Release can, however, be induced by treatment with the orally active hypoglycaemic agents referred to as the sulphonylureas, represented by chlorpropamide (see Table 12). The sulphonylureas are most effective in mature patients who are already stabilized on low doses of insulin, or who do not respond to purely dietary control. Patients receiving less than 20 units of insulin daily can usually be transferred directly to an oral drug, but in other cases the transfer should be carried out over a few days. For those patients who do not respond to the sulphonylureas, an alternative is the biguanide metformin. The mode of action differs, as it functions mainly by increasing the peripheral utilization of glucose. Guar gum has some antidiabetic properties, possibly mediated by interfering with the absorption of carbohydrates, and may be a useful supplementary treatment. Oral therapy with any antidiabetic drug is not suitable for juvenile or unstable diabetics.

Table 11. Insulin products

Product	Brand or other name	Origin	Approximate duration of action in hrs
Short-acting			
Soluble insulin	Soluble	beef	5–8
	Human Actrapid	H-pyr	
	Human Velosulin	H-emp	
	Humulin S	H-prb	
	Hypurin Neutral	beef	
	Velosulin	pork	
Intermediate acting			
Insulin Zinc (IZS) (amorphous)	Semitard MC	pork	18–24
	Human Initard	H-emp	
	Human Mixtard	H-emp	
Insulin Isophane (NPH + Soluble)	Humulin M1–4	H-prb	
	Initard	pork	
	Mixtard	pork	
Isophane insulin (NPH)	Isophane	pork	18–24
	Human Insulatard	H-emp	
	Human Protophane	H-pyr	
	Humulin I	H-prb	
	Insulatard	pork	
Long-acting			
Insulin Zinc Suspension (IZS) (amorphous + crystalline)	Human Monotard	H-pyr	18–30
	Hypurin Lente	beef	
	Lentard MC	pork and beef	
	Human Lente	H-prb	
Insulin Zinc Suspension (IZS) (crystalline)	Human Ultratard	H-pyr	24–28
	Humulin Zn	H-prb	
Protamine Zinc Insulin (P21)	Hypurin Protamine Zinc	beef	24–36

Product	Brand or other name	Origin	Approximate duration of action in hrs
Biphasic insulins	Initard 50/50%	pork	Mixture of insulins of varying duration of activity
	Mixtard 30/70%	pork	
	Human Actraphane 70/30%	H-pyr	
	Human Initard 50/50%	H-emp	
	Human Mixtard 70/30%	H-emp	
	Humulin M1 90/10%	H-prb	
	Humulin M2 80/20%	H-prb	
	Humulin M3 70/30%	H-prb	
	Humulin M4 60/40%	H-prb	
	Lentard MC	pork and beef	
	Rapitard MC	beef and pork	

Note: Human type insulins are prepared from enzyme modified pork insulin (emp), or by pro-insulin recombinant biosynthesis (prb), or via precursor yeast DNA technology (pyr).

Table 12. Anti-diabetic drugs

Approved names	Brand names
sulphonylureas	
chlorpropamide	Diabinase
glibenclamide	Daonil, Semi-Daonil, Euglucon
gliclizide	Diamicron
glipizide	Glibenese, Minodiab
gliquodine	Glurenorm
tolazamide	Tolanase
tolbutamide	Rastinon
biguanide	
metformin	Glucophage, Orabet
others	
guar gum	Glucotard, Guarem, Guarina

Dysmenorrhoea

The pain of dysmenorrhoea is thought to result from uterine contractions, and mild analgesics may be of some value, as may antispasmodics such as alverine. As the contractions appear to be mediated by prostaglandins, drugs that inhibit the enzymes associated with prostaglandin production may be of more value in spasmodic dysmenorrhoea. Such drugs are represented by naproxen and related compounds used in the rheumatoid conditions (see page 214) which are best given before the onset, and continued during menstruation. In other cases suppression of ovulation by progestogens may be effective, as may mixed progestogen/oestrogen preparations.

Table 13. Drugs used to treat dysmenorrhoea

Approved names	Brand names
alverine	Spasmonal
naproxen	Naprosyn
hormones	
dydrogesterone	Duphaston
norethisterone	Primolut N, Utovlan
progestogen/oestrogen	Controvlar

Epilepsy

Epilepsy is a condition characterized by convulsions, popularly known as fits, which are the result of excessive stimulation of the brain by a variety of factors. The convulsions may vary from generalized seizures (*grand mal*); absence seizures with a transient loss of consciousness that may pass in a fraction of a second almost like a daydream; and localized epilepsy without loss of awareness, that may sometimes appear more like a change of mood (*petit mal*). No single drug is yet available that can control all types of seizures, but for many years phenobarbitone was the standard treatment. Related drugs such as methyphenobarbitone and primidone appear to owe their action to conversion in the body to phenobarbitone, and they all have sedative side-effects. For grand mal, phenytoin is often a first choice drug, but careful control of dose is necessary, and carbamazepine has a wider range of safety. Ethosuximide is used mainly in *petit mal*. Sodium valproate is effective in most types of epilepsy and some benzodiazepines are also of value as anticonvulsants. A new anti-epileptic drug with a more selective mode of action is vigabatrin. Epilepsy appears to be linked with a deficiency of the brain neurotransmitter GABA (gamma-aminobutyric acid). Vigabatrin inhibits the activity of the GABA-metabolizing enzyme, and so permits a rise in the brain level of GABA. At present, vigabatrin is used mainly in the treatment of epilepsy not responding to other drugs. In all cases, any change in treatment should be carried out slowly to prevent the precipitation of rebound seizures. Those drugs used by injection for the control of status epilepticus are indicated thus *.

Table 14. Anticonvulsants

Approved name	Brand name
Those effective in petit mal:	
phenobarbitone	Luminal
methylphenobarbitone	Prominal
clonazepam	Rivotril
ethosuximide	Emeside, Zarontin
sodium valproate	Epilim
Those effective in grand mal and other types of seizure:	
phenobarbitone	Luminal
methylphenobarbitone	Prominal
carbamazepine	Tegretol
chlormethiazole*	Heminevrin
clonazepam*	Rivotril
diazepam*	Diazemuls, Valium
lamotrigine	Lamictal
lorazepam*	Almazine, Ativan
phenytoin*	Epanutin
primidone	Mysoline
sodium valproate	Epilim
vigabatrin	Sabril

*Indicates those drugs used in status epilepticus.

Heart failure

Heart failure is an inability of the heart to meet all the normal physiological demands of the body. In the early stages heart failure may be noted only on exercise, when the reduction in cardiac efficiency causes shortness of breath. As the condition progresses the heart fails to empty completely, so blood accumulates in the heart, and the back-pressure thus set up leads to further breathlessness, with congestion of the lungs and fluid accumulation which leads to ankle oedema. Basically, treatment is aimed at breaking the vicious circle of heart failure-congestion-oedema-increasing heart weakness. For mild heart failure, without marked pulmonary oedema, first-line treatment is with a thiazide diuretic, such as bendrofluazide, which by reducing the volume of fluid in the circulation, relieves the cardiac work-load and improves the cardiac efficiency (see Table 15). Some of the vasodilatory drugs used in the treatment of hypertension (see page 199) are also of value in heart failure, as the vasodilatation they produce lowers the peripheral resistance and so improves cardiac output. In more severe heart failure, digoxin, the glycoside of the foxglove, remains the drug of choice. It has a selective stimulatory action on the myocardium, resulting in more powerful and efficient contractions of the heart muscle, and improves the general circulation. Digoxin also acts on the vagus nerve and reduces the heart rate, and with increased cardiac efficiency the myocardial oxygen demand is reduced. The improvement in the circulation also promotes renal efficiency and relieves the oedema. Lanatoside has a similar action. A class of drugs of increasing importance in the treatment of heart failure are the angiotensin-converting enzyme inhibitors (ACE inhibitors). They are used in conjunction with diuretics and digoxin. Enoximone and milrinone are enzyme inhibitors that have a digoxin-like action on the myocardium, and are used in congestive heart failure not responding to other drugs. Xamoterol is a sympathomometic agent used only in exercise-induced mild heart failure. It should be withdrawn if the condition deteriorates.

Table 15. Drugs used to treat heart failure

Approved names	**Brand names**
diuretics	
bendrofluazide	Aprinox, Berkozide, Centyl, Neo-Naclex
See also page 200	
cardiac glycosides	
digoxin	Lanoxin, Lanoxin-PG
lanatoside C	Cedilanid
ACE inhibitors	
captopril*	Acepril, Capoten
cilazapril	Vascase
enalapril	Innovace
fosinopril	Staril
lisinopril	Carace, Zestril
quinapril	Accupro
ramipril	Tritase
others	
enoximone	Perfan
milrinone	Primacor
prazocin	Hypovase
xamoterol	Corwin
See also page 199	

*Acezide and Capozide are mixed products containing captopril and hydrochlorothiazide.

Herpes simplex

Herpes simplex or cold sore is a recurrent viral infection, which appears as a small cluster of vesicles, filled with clear fluid in an inflamed area. It usually appears on the lips and mucosa, but genital herpes can also occur. (Herpes simplex keratitis is a viral infection of the eye.) Herpes zoster is a related but more severe skin condition. Treatment is with antiviral drugs such as idoxuridine or acyclovir applied locally, but acyclovir is also given orally, usually as a 5-day course of treatment. In severe and systemic infections, it is given by intravenous infusion. In immunocompromised patients, acyclovir is given orally for long-term prophylaxis. Inosine pranobex is also used orally in the treatment of superficial herpes, and as auxiliary therapy in genital warts.
Note: Zidovudine is an antiviral drug effective against the AIDS virus: ganciclovir is used in infections due to the cytomegalovirus.

Table 16. Drugs used to treat herpes simplex

Approved names	Brand names
acyclovir	Zovirax
idoxuridine	Herpid 5%
	Iduridin (5% and 40%) in dimethyl sulphoxide
	Virudox (5%)
	Idoxene (0.5%) (Ophthalmic)
	Kerecid (0.5%)
inosine pranobex	Imunovir
ganciclovir	Cymevene
zidovudine	Retrovir

Hyperlipidaemia

Coronary atherosclerosis and associated conditions are linked with a high plasma level of cholesterol and triglycerides. Those plasma lipids are not present as such, as they are protein bound, and circulate as macromolecular complexes termed lipoproteins. They can be divided into very low density lipoproteins (VLDL), low-density lipoproteins (LDL) and a very high-density fraction (VHDL). Most of the plasma cholesterol is transported by LDL, and a high level of LDL is associated with increased cardiovascular risks. High levels of LDL can be reduced to some extent by a low-fat diet, but therapy by the use of plasma lipid-lowering drugs is often required. Nicotinic acid reduces the formation of LDL in the liver, but the high doses necessary, up to 3g daily, cause marked peripheral vasodilatation, a side-effect that makes the drug unacceptable by many patients. Nicofuranose and acipimox, which are derivatives of nicotinic acid, have a similar but less intense vasodilatory action. Probucol, an unrelated compound, appears to act at an early stage of cholesterol synthesis, and to promote the clearance of LDL, and fish oil lowers triglyceride levels, but reliance is largely placed on the use of ion-exchange resins, represented by cholestyramine, and on drugs of the clofibrate group. The exchange resins bind bile acids in the intestines, and interrupt the enterohepatic circulation of bile acids by preventing their re-absorption. The metabolic synthesis of cholesterol from bile acids is thus indirectly inhibited. That inhibition leads to a mobilization of cholesterol from stores in the liver, or withdrawal from cholesterol-containing LDL. The result is a slow lowering of both cholesterol and LDL plasma levels, but prolonged treatment is necessary.

Clofibrate and similar drugs reduce plasma triglyceride levels by stimulating the enzyme lipoprotein lipase. They also reduce cholesterol levels, but to a lesser extent. The side-effects of the clofibrate group include nausea and abdominal discomfort and care is necessary in renal impairment. Clofibrate increases biliary excretion of cholesterol, and accelerates gallstone formation. With gemfibrozil, blood and liver function tests should be carried out before and during treatment. A new approach to the problem of hyperlipidaemia is the use of selective enzyme inhibitors.

Cholesterol is synthesized to a great extent in the liver, and one of the enzymes concerned in that complex process is referred to as HMG-CoA reductase. Simvastatin and pravastatin are inhibitors of that enzyme, and so prevent further cholesterol synthesis. Plasma levels of cholesterol are maintained by drawing on reserves in the liver, and as those reserves dwindle, the plasma levels of cholesterol gradually fall. These drugs are used in hyperlipidaemia not responding to other therapy, and as extended treatment is necessary, liver function tests should be carried out at intervals of 4–6 weeks. Side-effects are constipation, nausea, abdominal pain, rash and diarrhoea.

Table 17. Antihyperlipidaemic drugs

Approved name	Brand name	Daily dose
Nicotinic acid and derivatives		
nicotinic acid		1–6g
acipimox	Olbetam	500–750mg
nicofuranose	Bradilan	1–3g
Exchange resins		
cholestyramine	Questran	12–24g
colestipol	Colestid	10–30g
Clofibrate and similar drugs		
bezafibrate	Bezalip	600mg
clofibrate	Atromid-S	2g
fenofibrate	Lipantil	300mg
gemfibrozil	Lopid	1–1.5g
Enzyme inhibitors		
simvastatin	Zocor	10–40mg
pravastatin	Lipostat	10–40mg
Others		
probucol	Lurselle	1g
fish oil	Maxepa	10g

Hypertension

Hypertension is a state of continued high blood pressure. Essential hypertension is of no known or obvious cause, and is often linked with age. Secondary hypertension may be caused by renal disease, pregnancy or rarely by an adrenaline-producing tumour (phaeochromocytoma). Treatment is aimed at reducing the elevated blood pressure to a level consistent with the age and condition of the patient, and not to an artificially low level that might reduce the blood supply to essential organs such as the kidneys. The range of drugs used in hypertension is extensive and combined therapy with drugs that act at different points may give the best overall control.

Beta-adrenoceptor blocking agents (beta-blockers) of which propranolol is one of many, are in wide use (see Table 18), and are often given in association with thiazide diuretics (see bendrofluazide and Table 18). The calcium channel blocking agents used in angina are also effective in hypertension, but are indicated mainly in patients not responding to other therapy. Another approach to the treatment of hypertension is the use of angiotensin-converting enzyme inhibitors (ACE inhibitors). These drugs act by inhibiting the formation of angiotensin II, the most powerful natural pressor substance, and are highly effective as blood pressure lowering agents. They also have applications in the treatment of heart failure. In general they are well tolerated, but initial therapy requires care, as they bring about a marked first-dose fall in blood pressure, and a first dose should be taken at night with the patient in bed. Other antihypertensive drugs act by blocking alpha-adrenoceptors, and may also cause a first-dose hypotension. Other drugs in less frequent use are represented by clonidine, methyldopa, bethanidine, debrisoquine, guanethidine, hydralazine and reserpine. Minoxidil is given in severe hypertension resistant to other drugs; diazoxide and sodium nitroprusside are given intravenously in the control of hypertensive crisis.

Table 18. Antihypertensive drugs

Approved names	Brand names
Beta-adrenoceptor blocking agents (beta-blockers)	
acebutolol	Sectral
atenolol	Tenormin
betaxolol	Kerlone
bisoprolol	Emcor, Monocor
esmolol	Brevibloc
labetalol	Trandate
metoprolol	Betaloc, Lopressor, Betaloc SA*, Lopresor SR*, Meteros*, Meteros LS*
nadolol	Corgard
oxprenolol	Trasicor, Slow-Pren*, Slow-Trasicor*
pindodol	Betadren, Visken
sotolol	Beta-Cardone, Sotacor
timolol	Betim, Blocadren
	*Long-acting products
Thiazide and other diuretics	
amiloride**	Midamor
bendrofluazide	Aprinox; Berkozide; Centyl; Neo-Naclex
bumetanide*	Burinex
carenoate***	Spiroctan-M
chlorothiazide	Saluric
chlorthalidone	Hygroton
cyclopenthiazide	Navidrex
ethacrynic acid*	Edecrin
frusemide*	Aluzine; Diuresal; Dryptal; Lasix
hydrochlorothiazide	Esidrex; HydroSaluric
hydroflumethiazide	Hydrenox
indapamide	Natrilix
mefruside	Baycaron
methyclothiazide	Enduron
metolazone	Netinex S
piretanide*	Arelix
polythiazide	Nephril
spironolactone***	Aldactone; Diatensic; Laractone; Spiroctan; Spiriolone
triamterene	Dytac
xipamide	Diurexan
*loop	
**potassium-sparing	
***aldosterone antagonists	
calcium channel blocking agents	
diltiazem	Britiazem, Tildiem

Approved names	Brand names
felodipine	Plendil
isradipine	Prescal
nicardipine	Cardone
nifedipine	Adalat, Adalat Retard*, Adalate IC (injection)
nimodipine	Nimotop
verapamil	Berkatens, Cordilox, Securon, Securon SR*, Univer*
	*Sustained release
ACE inhibitors	
captopril	Acepril, Capoten
cilazapril	Vascase
enalapril	Innovace
fosinopril	Staril
lisinopril	Carace, Zestril
perindopril	Coversyl
quinapril	Accupro
ramipril	Tritace
*Acezide and Capozide contain captopril and hydrochlorthiazide	
others	
bethanidine	Bendogen, Esbatal
clonidine	Catapres
debrisoquine	Declinax
diazoxide	Eudemine
doxazocin	Cardura
guanethidine	Ismelin
hydralazine	Apresoline
indoramin	Baratol
methyldopa	Aldomet, Dopamet
minoxodil	Loniten
phenoxybenzamine	Dibenyline
phentolamine	Rogitine
prazocin	Hypovase
reserpine	Serpasil
sodium nitroprousside	Nipride
terazocin	Hytrin

Insomnia

Insomnia is a common condition, and with advancing age the total sleep period tends to shorten, and become more interrupted. It is sometimes more apparent than real, as although insomniacs may have a disturbed sleep pattern, they may in fact sleep more than they realize. Initial insomnia, or difficulty in falling asleep, may be due to anxiety, whereas early morning awakening, after which the individual finds difficulty in falling asleep again, may be associated with depression, or be merely part of the ageing process. In all cases, before any treatment is instituted, any underlying cause of the insomnia such as cough or pain should be dealt with, and any stimulants should be avoided. The drugs used to treat insomnia include sedatives and hypnotics. Sedatives reduce mental activity and pre-dispose to sleep, whereas hypnotics are sleep-inducing drugs, but there is no sharp distinction, as small doses of hypnotics may have a useful sedative effect. Barbiturates were once widely used as hypnotics, and although some are still available, tolerance and dependence may easily occur. Their use has declined sharply since the introduction of the hypnotic benzodiazepines represented by nitrazepam. These drugs are suitable for the short-term treatment of insomnia, and are best given about 30 min before bedtime. Some have a longer action than others, and may have hangover effects, and with extended treatment may have a cumulative action. Chloral is a time-honoured hypnotic which is also suitable in small doses for children; triclofos is a chloral derivative. Promethazine is an antihistamine that is also used as a mild hypnotic. Chlormethiazole is more suitable for elderly patients as it has few after-effects, and zopiclone is a new unrelated hypnotic. Any treatment with an hypnotic should be withdrawn slowly to reduce any rebound insomnia.

Table 19. Hypnotics

Approved names	Brand names	Daily dose range
Benzodiazepines		
flunitrazepam	Rohypnol	0.5–2mg
flurazepam	Dalmane	15–30mg
loprazolam		1–2mg
lormetazepam		0.5–1.5mg
nitrazepam	Mogadon, Somnite, Surem, Unisomnia	5–10mg
temazepam[a]	Normisan	10–60mg
triazolam[a]	Halcion	0.25mg
Other hypnotics		
chloral hydrate	Notec	0.5–2g
chloral betaine	Welldorm	0.5–2g
chlormethiazole	Heminevrin	192–384mg
promethazine	Phenergan,Sominex	25–50mg
zoplicone	Zimovane	7.5–15mg

[a]short-acting hypnotics

Migraine

Migraine is an episodic condition characterized by severe headache, visual disturbances, nausea and vomiting. The flashes of light that occur may be due to cerebral vasoconstriction, but the headache is thought to be linked with vasodilatation of the cranial arteries. The cause is unknown, but some apparently innocuous dietary products such as chocolate or cheese may initiate an attack, and oral contraceptives may both precipitate migraine and increase the severity of an established attack. Some cases of migraine may respond to simple analgesics like aspirin and paracetamol, but more potent treatment is usually required. Ergotamine is often the first choice, as it constricts the cranial arteries, but it has little effect on the visual disturbances, and may even increase the nausea and vomiting, and require anti-emetic therapy (see page 208). When vomiting is a problem, ergotamine can be given by aerosol inhalation or by suppository. Isometheptene is a sympathometic agent and has vasoconstrictor properties that is also used in the treatment of migraine.

Dihydroergotamine is an alternative drug given by injection in patients not responding to other treatment. For the prophylatic treatment of migraine reliance is often placed on pizotifen, which has some antiserotonin and anti-histaminic properties, but it may bring about an increase in weight. Cyproheptadyne has similar properties and uses. Beta-blockers are also used in the prophylaxis of migraine, and the use of a long-acting product may permit a single daily dose (see page 200). Clonidine, which is used in hypertension, is also given in small doses for migraine prophylaxis. Methysergide is used in the prophylaxis of very severe migraine not responding to other drugs, but it may cause fibrotic reactions, and is used only under hospital supervision.

More recently, it has become clear that serotonin (5HT) has a more specific action in bringing about cranial vasoconstriction, an effect mediated via the $5HT_1$ – like receptors. A serotonin analogue with a selective action on those receptors is sumatriptan. It is given in doses of 6mg by subcutaneous injection via an auto-injection device as soon as possible after an attack of migraine has begun, when it gives rapid relief of migraine and cluster headache. A second dose if required may be given after 1 hour up to a maximum dose of 12mg in 24 hrs. Like ergotamine, sumatriptan is not suitable for prophylaxis.

Table 20. Drugs used to treat migraine

Approved names	Brand names
ergotamine	Cafergot*, Lingraine, Migril*, Medihaler-Ergotamine
dihydroergotamine	Dihydergot
isometheptene	Midrid*
clonidine	Dixarit
cyproheptadine	Periactin
methysergide	Deseril
pizotifen	Sanomigran
sumatriptan	Imigran

*These are mixed products with supplementary drugs such as caffeine or paracetamol.

Migraleve, Migraves and Faramax are anti-emetic products containing metoclopramide with a mild analgesic.

Myocardial infarction

Myocardial infarction, often referred to as coronary thrombosis or a heart attack, is a sudden reduction in the flow of blood to part of the myocardium, and is associated with the presence of a blood clot. It is characterized by a severe and prolonged angina-like pain and cardiac arrhythmias. The pain is seldom relieved by glyceryl trinitrate (unlike angina pectoris), and injections of morphine, buprenorphine or a similar powerful analgesic may be required, but remedial treatment is with a fibrinolytic agent, given as soon as possible by intravenous injection. Other treatment is with drugs of the lignocaine type to control the cardiac arrhythmias, together with digoxin and diuretics for the heart failure. Subsequent long-term control involves the use of beta-blockers, specific anti-arrhythmic agents, lipid-lowering drugs*, exchange resins, enzyme inhibitors, platelet stabilizers and anticoagulants.

*See Hyperlipidaemia

Table 21. Drugs used to treat myocardial infarction

Approved names	Brand names
Analgesics	
buprenorphine	Temegesic
Fibrinolytic agents	
alteplase	Actilase
anistreplase	Eminase
streptokinase	Kabikinase, Streptase
urokinase	Ukidan, Urokinase
Anti-arrhythmics	
disopyramide	Rythmodan
flecainide	Tambocor
lignocaine	Xylocard
Beta-blockers	
metoprolol	Betaloc, Lopresor
mexiletine	Mexitil
propranolol	Inderal, Slopropol, Apsolol, Berkolol, Cardinol, Angilol
timolol	Betim, Blocadren
Platelet stabilizers	
aspirin	Angettes, Platet
dipyridamole	Persantin
Lipid lowering agents	
bezafibrate	Bezalip
clofibrate	Atromid-S
fenofibrate	Lipantil
gemfibrozil	Lopid
Exchange resins	
cholestyramine	Questran, Questran-A
colestipol	Colestid
Enzyme inhibitors	
probucol	Lurselle
simvastatin	Zocor
pravastatin	Lipostat
Anticoagulants	
nicoumalone	Sinthrome
phenindione	Dindevan
warfarin	Marevan

Nausea and vomiting

Nausea and vomiting can be triggered off by a number of factors, ranging from gastric irritation, including that caused by drugs, disturbances of balance such as vertigo, or by pregnancy and travelling. The condition is ultimately linked with a stimulation of the vomiting centre in the brain, and most anti-emetics function by an action on that centre. The alkaloid hyoscine is widely used in travel sickness, as are the antihistamines, and for the best results should be taken prophylactically before a journey. As an alternative to oral therapy, a skin patch containing hyoscine may be used to obtain an extended action. Many of these anti-emetics have sedative side-effects, and they should not be used routinely in the vomiting of pregnancy. Some antipsychotic agents of the chlorpromazine type have a more selective action, as they are dopamine antagonists, and have a blocking action on the chemoreceptor trigger zone of the vomiting centre. Domperidone and nabilone are other powerful anti-emetics with similar uses.

It has long been known that the vomiting reflex is stimulated by the release of serotonin in the gut, and metoclopramide has an anti-emetic action, mediated in part at least, by serotonin blockade. It is given in high doses in the severe nausea and vomiting caused by chemotherapeutic agents in the treatment of cancer where the nausea may be so intense that patients may refuse further treatment. Recently it has been shown that a sub-group of serotonin receptors (the $5HT_3$ receptors) is linked with the initiation of the vomiting reflex. Two specific drugs for the blockade of $5HT_3$ receptors are now available, ondansetron and granisetron, and their introduction has opened a new approach to the problem of controlling the severe nausea and vomiting in patients receiving high doses of cyclophosphamide and similar drugs, in bone marrow transplants and other conditions associated with severe nausea and vomiting.

Table 22. Anti-emetics

Approved names	Brand names
hyoscine	Scopoderm TS (skin patch)
Antihistamines	
cinnarizine	Stugeron
cyclizine	Valoid
dimenhydrinate	Dramamine
promethazine	Phenergan
promethazine theoclate	Avomine
Chlorpromazine group	
chlorpromazine	Largactil
perphenazine	Fentazin
	Buccastem
prochlorperazine	Stemetil
	Vertigon
thiethylperazine	Torecan
Others	
granisetron	Kytril
metoclopramide	Gastromax
	Maxolon
nabilone	Cesamet
ondansetron	Zofran

Parkinsonism

Parkinsonism is a degenerative disease associated with a progressive reduction in the amount of dopamine, a neurotransmitter substance, formed in the substantia nigra of the brain. As a result, the normal balance between the brain levels of dopamine and acetylcholine is disturbed, and is the basic cause of the tremor, muscular rigidity and slowness characteristic of parkinsonism. For many years the only treatment was with anticholinergic agents, and they remain of value in controlling the rigidity and tremor of mild forms of the illness. Amantadine is an unrelated drug with reduced side-effects, but some patients may fail to respond, and tolerance may limit its value. Although parkinsonism is due to a dopamine deficiency, dopamine cannot be given directly as replacement therapy as it is poorly absorbed, and does not cross the blood brain barrier, and its amino acid precursor, levodopa, although better absorbed, is inactivated to some extent by liver enzymes, and so fails to reach the brain in a fully effective concentration. The problem can be overcome by giving levodopa together with a specific inhibitor such as benserazide or carbidopa. The combination permits a larger amount of levodopa to reach the brain where it is converted to active dopamine. Additional therapy with an anticholinergic agent may improve the response, and in some cases permit a reduction in the "end-of-dose" loss of symptomatic control. Selegiline acts upon another enzyme, and is given together with levodopa in severe parkinsonism. Bromocriptine is a secondary drug that appears to act by stimulating any surviving dopamine receptors in the brain, but side-effects may limit its value. Lysuride is a new drug with a similar stimulatory action.

Pergolide is another new dopamine agonist that acts on both D_1 and D_2 receptors. Combined treatment with these auxilliary drugs, and careful adjustment of doses, including those of levodopa, may improve the overall response, reduce the severity of side-effects, and possibly delay further deterioration of the patient's condition.

Table 23. Anti-parkinsonism drugs

Approved names	Brand names
Anticholinergic agents	
benzhexol	Artane, Bentex, Broflex
benztropine	Cogentin
biperidon	Akineton
methixine	Tremonil
orphenadrine	Biorphen, Disipal
procyclidine	Arpicolin, Kemadrin
Levodopa and mixed products	
levodopa	Brocadopa, Larodopa
co-beneldopa (levodopa with benserazide)	Madopar
co-careldopa (levodopa with carbidopa)	Sinamet
Others	
amantadine	Mantadine, Symmetrel
bromocriptine	Parlodel
lysuride	Revanil
selegiline	Eldepryl

Peptic Ulcer

The term peptic ulcer includes gastric ulcer, duodenal ulcer and the less common oesophageal ulcers. It is a medical axiom that 'no acid – no ulcer', and for many years gastric ulcers were treated with antacids such as magnesium trisilicate. Bismuth chelate has a protective action by coating the ulcerated areas, whereas sulcralfate appears to act by protecting the gastric mucosa from acid-pepsin attack. Acid secretion can be suppressed by anti-cholinergic agents, and pirenzepine has a relatively selective action on gastric acid secretion. Misoprostol is a prostaglandin analogue which also inhibits gastric acid secretion, and it is also of value in the prophylaxis of peptic ulcers induced by NSAIDs. Carbenoxolone has a chemical relationship with a constituent of liquorice, and has some ulcer-healing properties. It appears to have a protective action by increasing the production of mucin. In recent years, reliance has been placed to an increasing extent on the histamine H_2-receptor blocking agents, which have a selective inhibitory action on gastric acid secretion, and so promote the healing of peptic ulcers by a more direct attack on the initial cause. Extended treatment with intermittent rest periods is necessary to avoid relapse. Omeprazole acts in a different manner by inhibiting an enzyme at a later stage of acid formation, and is effective in the treatment of ulcers resistant to other drugs.

Table 24. Anti-ulcer drugs

Approved names	Brand names
bismuth chelate	De-nol, De-Noltab
sucralfate	Antepsin
misoprostol	Cytotec
pirenzepine	Gastrozepin
carbenoxolone	Biogastrone
H_2-receptor blocking agents	
cimetidine	Dyspamet, Tagamet, Algitec
famotidine	Pepcid PM
nizatidine	Axid
ranitidine	Zantac
Enzyme inhibitor	
omeprazole	Losec

Rheumatoid and osteoarthritis

Rheumatoid arthritis is a chronic inflammatory disease of the joints with local swelling and pain. The cause is unknown, and although partial remission and exacerbations occur, the disease is a progressive one, and in severe conditions bed-rest may be necessary. In osteoarthritis, degeneration of the joints also occurs. Treatment is largely symptomatic, and is based on the non-steroidal anti-inflammatory drugs (NSAIDS) of which aspirin is the oldest and one of the most widely used. The NSAIDS have analgesic as well as anti-inflammatory properties, and act by suppressing the production of inflammatory prostaglandins. The choice of a NSAID depends much upon individual response, as they are potential gastric irritants, and are best taken after food. Patients vary widely in their tolerance to any particular NSAID, and they have many side-effects. To obtain prolonged relief at night, and to reduce morning stiffness, some NSAIDS are available as suppositories. Corticosteroids are also used mainly in conditions not responding to NSAIDS, and are sometimes given by direct injection into a joint. In some cases of rheumatoid arthritis, the progression of the disease can be halted for a time by drugs that modify the underlying degenerative process, as with gold salts, penicillamine, and less frequently chloroquine and salazopyrine. Sodium aurothiomalate is a gold compound given by injection, but auranofin is an orally active gold preparation. Some immunosuppressive drugs such as azothiaprine have an action similar to that of the gold compounds. The use of all these disease-modifying drugs requires great care.

Table 25. Drugs used to treat arthritis

Approved names	Brand names
Non-steroidal anti-inflammatory drugs (NSAIDs)	
acetmetacin	Emflex
azapropazone	Rheumox
benorylate	Benoral
*diclofenac	Rheumalgan, Voltarol
etodolac	Lodine
fenbrufen	Lederfen
fenoprofen	Fenopron, Progesic
flurbiprofen	Froben
ibuprofen	Apsifen, Brufen, Fenbid, Ibular, Lidofen, Motrin, Paxofen
*indomethacin	Flexin, Imbrilon, Indocid, Indolar, Indomed, Mobilan, Rheumacin, SloIndo
*ketoprofen	Alrheumat, Orudis, Orivail
mefenamic acid	Ponstan
nabumetone	Relifex
*naproxen	Laraflex, Naprosyn, Synflex
*piroxicam	Feldene, Larapam
salsalate	Disalcid
sulindac	Clinoril
tenoxicam	Mobilflex
tiaprofenic acid	Surgam
tolmetin	Tolectin
Gold compounds	
sodium aurothiomalate	Myocrisin
auranofin	Ridura
Others	
penicillamine	Distamine, Pendramine
chloroquine	Avloclor, Nivaquine
salazopyrine	Salazopyrin
Immunosuppressants	
azathioprine	Azamune, Berkaprine, Imuran
chlorambucil	Leukeran
cyclophosphamide	Endoxana
methotrexate	Maxtrex

*also available as suppositories

Schizophrenia

Schizophrenia is a serious mental disorder, with hallucinations and delusions, a deterioration in thought patterns and reasoning ability, and an increasing disability to distinguish between the imaginary and the real. It may develop slowly, or be a rapid response to stress. In some patients a condition of apathy and withdrawal may be the most prominent symptom. The range of anti-psychotic drugs used in the treatment of schizophrenia is wide and extending, as new types of drugs are introduced. The drugs in most frequent use are phenothiazines of the chlorpromazine type, referred to as either anti-psychotic drugs or major tranquillizers. The different members of the group exhibit certain differences in action, as some may be more effective in controlling the most marked symptoms of schizophrenia, and others may be of more value in apathetic patients, but the distinction is not sharp. In all cases, prolonged treatment is essential, as improvement may be slow, and drug withdrawal should be correspondingly slow, as relapse may occur. Schizophrenia is considered to be due to an imbalance of certain factors in the brain, and many anti-psychotic drugs act by blocking dopamine receptors, thus permitting a rise in the brain level of dopamine. That rise may be associated with some of the side-effects of the chlorpromazine group of drugs. In some cases, improvement once achieved can be maintained by the use of long-acting depot injections of the drug concerned, which reduce to some extent the problems of patient compliance with therapy.

Many other anti-psychotic drugs unrelated to chlorpromazine have a basically similar action. Sulpiride is exceptional, as in high doses it can control the more severe forms of schizophrenia, whereas in small doses it has an altering effect on withdrawn patients.

Table 26. Drugs used to treat schizophrenia

Approved names	**Brand names**
Sedative phenothiazines	
chlorpromazine	Largactil
promazine	Sparine
methotrimeprazine	Nozinan
Less sedative phenothiazines	
pericyazine	Neulactil
pipothiazine	Piportil
thioridazine	Melleril
Phenothiazines with increased extra-pyramidal side-effects	
fluphenazine	Moditen
perphenazine	Fentazin
prochlorperazine	Stemetil, Buccastem
trifluoperazine	Stelazine
Other antischizophrenics	
clozapine	Clozaril
flupenthixol	Depixol
fluspirilene	Redeptin
haloperidol	Dozic, Fortunan, Haldol, Serenace
loxapine	Loxapac
oxypertine	Integrin
pimozide	Orap
remoxipride	Roxiam
sulpiride	Dolmatil, Sulpitil
trifluoperidol	Triperidol

Ulcerative colitis

Ulcerative colitis is an abnormal condition of the lower intestinal tract, particularly the colon, and is characterized by a breakdown of the mucosal layer with inflammation and ulceration, and attacks of bloody diarrhoea, abdominal pain and dehydration. Remission and recurrence may occur without apparent cause. As the disease progresses, the muscular coat of the intestines may be involved, with further ulceration. Crohn's disease is very similar, but may affect other parts of the intestinal tract. Mild conditions may respond to codeine, but more specific treatment is with sulphasalazine and prednisolone, which may be given orally or as retention enemas, and less frequently azathiaprine is given. Sulphasalazine has certain side-effects associated with the 'sulpha' part of the drug, and the derivatives mesalazine and olsalazine may be better tolerated.

Table 27. Drugs used to treat ulcerative colitis

Approved names	Brand names
sulphasalazine	Salazopyrin
mesalazine	Asacol, Pentasa
olsalazine	Dipentum, Azamune, Berkaprine
azathioprine	Imuran
prednisolone	Deltacortril Enteric
	Deltastab
	Precortisyl
	Prenesol
	Sintisone
	*Predenema
	*Predfoam
	*Predsol
	*Rectal products

Urinary incontinence and frequency

Normal urinary control is the result of a complex process involving many factors, including the interaction of both smooth and voluntary muscle. Loss of that control may arise from a variety of causes, including a disturbance of the local nerve supply to the bladder, when the term neurogenic bladder is sometimes used, or it may arise from trauma or infection. Urinary incontinence is characterized by an involuntary passing of urine, which is preceded by an urgent desire to void. Stress incontinence is an uncontrollable loss of urine as a result of coughing, straining or any other activity that brings about a sudden increase in the intra-abdominal pressure. It is more common in women than in men.

Overflow incontinence usually occurs as the result of an obstruction, or of impaired detrusor muscle contraction. The bladder fills until the urinary pressure overcomes the sphincter resistance, and the urine then dribbles from the urethra, whereas frequency may be due to trauma, infection or inflammation. Nocturnal enuresis is the involuntary and periodic urination that occurs during sleep in children, and is more common in boys than in girls. For symptomatic treatment, reliance is based largely on the anticholinergic agents represented by propantheline. Such agents, including the recently introduced oxbutynin, inhibit the effects of acetycholine on smooth muscle, reduce erratic detrusor muscle contractions and increase stability. The use of certain tricyclic antidepressants in the treatment of frequency and urinary incontinence is also based on their anticholinergic action. Ephedrine is used mainly in enuresis, as it relaxes the bladder wall, contracts the sphincter, and relaxes the detrusor muscle. A few drugs, such as flavoxate, have a direct antispasmodic action. Desmopressin, an analogue of the pressor principle of the posterior pituitary gland, has also been used for the treatment of enuresis. Prostatic hypertrophy, by causing bladder outlet obstruction, may also cause urinary problems and incontinence. In such cases, alpha-receptor blocking agents may reduce bladder muscle tone and give symptomatic improvement, particularly in patients awaiting surgery.

Table 28. Drugs used in incontinence

Approved names	Brand names
Anticholinergic agents	
propantheline	Pro-Banthine
terodiline	Micturin
oxbutynin	Ditopan
Tricyclic antidepressants	
amitriptyline	Domical, Lentizol, Tryptizol
imipramine	Tofranil
nortriptyline	Concordin
Others	
ephedrine	
flavoxate	Urispas
desmopressin	DDAVP, Desmospray
Alpha-adrenoceptor blocking agents	
indoramin	Doralese
prazocin	Hypovase

Approved and proprietary names of drugs

Approved Name	Proprietary Name	Main action or Indication
acebutolol	Sectral	hypertension
acemetacin	Emflex	arthritis
acetazolamide	Diamox	glaucoma
acetylcysteine	Fabrol; Parvolex	mucolytic; paracetamol overdose
acipimox	Olbetam	hyperlipidaemia
aclarubicin	Aclacin	cytotoxic
acrivastine	Semprex	antihistamine
acrosoxacin	Eradacin	gonorrhoea
actinomycin D	Cosmegen	cytotoxic
acyclovir	Zovirax	antiviral
adenosine	Adenocor	paroxysmal tachycardia
alclomethasone	Modrasone	topical corticosteroid
alcuronium	Alloferin	muscle relaxant
alfacalcidol	One-Alpha	vitamin D deficiency
alfentanil	Rapifen	narcotic analgesic
allopurinol	Aloral; Aluline; Caplenal; Hamarin; Zyloric	gout
allyloestrenol	Gestanin	progestogen
almasilate	Malinal	antacid
aloxiprin	Palaprin	arthritis
alprazolam	Xanax	antidepressant
alprostadil	Prostin VR	maintenance of ductus arteriosus in neonates
alteplase	Actilyse	fibrinolytic
alverine	Spasmonal	antispasmodic
amantadine	Symmetrel	parkinsonism
amikacin	Amikin	antibiotic
amiloride	Midamor	diuretic
aminoglutethimide	Orimeten	cytotoxic
amiodarone	Cordarone	anti-arrhythmic
amitriptyline	Domical; Lentizol; Tryptizol	antidepressant
amlodipine	Istin	calcium antagonist
amorolfine	Loceryl	topical antifungal
amoxapine	Asendis	antidepressant
amoxycillin	Almodan; Amoxil	antibiotic
amphotericin B	Fungilin; Fungizone	antifungal

Approved Name	Proprietary Name	Main action or Indication
ampicillin	Amfipen; Penbritin; Vidopen	antibiotic
amsacrine	Amsidine	cytotoxic
amylobarbitone	Amytal	hypnotic
anistreplase	Eminase	fibrinolytic
aprotinin	Trasylol	haemostatic
astemizole	Hismanal	antihistamine
atenolol	Tenormin	beta-blocker
atracurium	Tracrium	muscle relaxant
auranofin	Ridaura	rheumatoid arthritis
azapropazone	Rheumox	antirheumatic
azatadine	Optimine	antihistamine
azathioprine	Azamune; Berkaprine; Imuran	immunosuppressive
azelastine	Rhinolast	topical antihistamine
azidothymidine	Retrovir	antiviral
azithromycin	Zithromax	antibiotic
azlocillin	Securopen	antibiotic
aztreonam	Azactam	antibiotic
bacampicillin	Ambaxin	antibiotic
baclofen	Lioresal	muscle relaxant
beclomethasone	Becotide Propaderm	corticosteroid topical corticosteroid
bendrofluazide	Aprinox; Berkozide; Centyl; Neo-Naclex	diuretic
benorylate	Benoral	analgesic
benperidol	Anquil	tranquillizer
benzalkonium chloride	Roccal	antiseptic
benzathine penicillin	Penidural	antibiotic
benzhexol	Artane; Bentex; Broflex	parkinsonism
benztropine	Cogentin	parkinsonism
benzylpenicillin	Crystapen	antibiotic
bephenium	Alcopar	anthelmintic
betahistine	Serc	Ménière's syndrome
betamethasone	Betnelan; Betnesol Betnovate	corticosteroid topical corticosteroid
betaxolol	Kerlone	beta-blocker

Approved Name	Proprietary Name	Main action or Indication
bethanechol	Myotonine	smooth muscle stimulant
bethanidine	Bendogen; Esbatal	hypertension
bezafibrate	Bezalip	hyperlipidaemia
biperiden	Akineton	parkinsonism
bisacodyl	Dulcolax	laxative
bisoprolol	Emcor; Monocor	beta-blocker
botulinum toxin	Dysport	blepharospasm
bretylium tosylate	Bretylate	cardiac arrhythmias
bromazepam	Lexotan	anxiolytic
bromocriptine	Parlodel	lactation suppressant
brompheniramine	Dimotane	antihistamine
budesonide	Pulmicort	asthma
	Rhinocort	rhinitis
bumetanide	Burinex	diuretic
bupivacaine	Marcaine	anaesthetic
buprenorphine	Temgesic	analgesic
buserelin	Suprefact	prostatic carcinoma
buspirone	Buspar	anxiolytic
busulphan	Myleran	cytotoxic
butobarbitone	Soneryl	hypnotic
butriptyline	Evadyne	antidepressant
cadexomer iodine	Iodosorb	leg ulcers
calcipotriol	Dovonex	psoriasis
calcitonin	Calcitare	hormone
calcitriol	Rocaltrol	vitamin D deficiency
canrenoate	Spiroctan-N	diuretic
capreomycin	Capastat	antibiotic
captopril	Acepril; Capoten	ACE inhibitor
carbamazepine	Tegretol	epilepsy
carbaryl	Carylderm; Derbac	parasiticide
carbenicillin	Pyopen	antibiotic
carbenoxolone	Biogastrone	peptic ulcer
carbimazole	Neo-Mercazole	thyrotoxicosis
carbocisteine	Mucodyne	mucolytic
carboplatin	Paraplatin	cytotoxic
carfecillin	Uticillin	antibiotic
carisoprodol	Carisoma	muscle relaxant
carmustine	BiCNU	cytotoxic
carteolol	Cartrol	beta-blocker
	Teoptic	glaucoma
cefaclor	Distaclor	antibiotic
cefadroxil	Baxan	antibiotic

Approved Name	Proprietary Name	Main action or Indication
cefixime	Suprax	antibiotic
cefotaxime	Claforan	antibiotic
cefoxitin	Nefoxin	antibiotic
cefsulodin	Monaspor	antibiotic
ceftazidime	Fortum	antibiotic
ceftizoxime	Cefizox	antibiotic
cefuroxime	Zinacef; Zinnat	antibiotic
celiprolol	Celectol	hypertension
cephalexin	Ceporex; Keflex	antibiotic
cephalothin	Keflin	antibiotic
cephamandole	Kefadol	antibiotic
cephazolin	Kefzol	antibiotic
cephradine	Velosef	antibiotic
cetirizine	Zirtek	antihistamine
chenodeoxycholic acid	Chendol; Chenofalk	gallstones
chloral betaine	Welldorm	hypnotic
chloral hydrate	Noctec	hypnotic
chlorambucil	Leukeran	cytotoxic
chloramphenicol	Chloromycetin; Kemicetine	antibiotic
chlordiazepoxide	Librium	anxiolytic
chlorhexidine	Hibitane	antiseptic
chlormethiazole	Heminevrin	hypnotic; anticonvulsant
chlormezanone	Trancopal	anxiolytic
chloroquine	Avloclor; Nivaquine	antimalarial
chlorothiazide	Saluric	diuretic
chlorpheniramine	Piriton	antihistamine
chlorpromazine	Largactil	tranquillizer
chlorpropamide	Diabinese	hypoglycaemic
chlortetracycline	Aureomycin	antibiotic
chlorthalidone	Hygroton	diuretic
cholestyramine	Questran	bile acid binder
choline theophyllinate	Choledyl; Sabidal	bronchodilator
cilazapril	Vascase	ACE inhibitor
cimetidine	Dyspamet; Tagamet	H_2-blocker
cinnarizine	Stugeron	anti-emetic
cinoxacin	Cinobac	antibiotic
ciprofloxacin	Ciproxin	antibacterial
cisapride	Alimix; Prepulsid	oesophageal reflux

Approved Name	Proprietary Name	Main action or Indication
clarithromycin	Klaricid	antibiotic
clemastine	Tavegil	antihistamine
clindamycin	Dalacin C	antibiotic
clobazam	Frisium	tranquillizer
clobetasol	Dermovate	topical corticosteroid
clobetasone	Eumovate	topical corticosteroid
clofazimine	Lamprene	antileprotic
clofibrate	Atromid S	hyperlipidaemia
clomiphene	Clomid; Serophene	infertility
clomipramine	Anafranil	antidepressant
clomocycline	Megaclor	antibiotic
clonazepam	Rivotril	epilepsy
clonidine	Catapres; Dixarit	hypertension; migraine
clorazepate	Tranxene	anxiolytic
clotrimazole	Canestan	antifungal
cloxacillin	Orbenin	antibiotic
clozapine	Clozaril	antipsychotic
co-amilofruse	Frumil; Lasoride	diuretic
co-amilozide	Amilco; Hypertane 50; Moduret 25; Moduretic; Normetic	diuretic
co-amoxiclav	Augmentin	antibiotic
co-beneldopa	Madopar	parkinsonism
co-careldopa	Sinemet	parkinsonism
co-codamol	Medocodone; Panadeine; Paracodol; Parake	analgesic
co-codaprin	Codis	analgesic
co-dergocrine	Hydergine	dementia
co-dydramol	Paramol	analgesic
co-fluampicil	Flu-Amp; Magnapen	antibiotic
co-flumactone	Aldactide	diuretic
colestipol	Colestid	exchange resin
colfosceril	Exosurf	neonatal respiratory distress
colistin	Colomycin	antibiotic
co-phenotrope	Lomotil	diarrhoea
co-prenozide	Trasidex	hypertension

Approved Name	Proprietary Name	Main action or Indication
co-proxamol	Cosalgesic; Distalgesic; Paxalgesic	analgesic
corticotrophin	Acthar	hormone
cortisone	Cortelan; Cortistab; Cortisyl	corticosteroid
co-simalcite	Altacite plus	antacid
co-tenidone	Tenoret 50; Tenoretic	hypertension
co-trimoxazole	Bactrim; Chemotrim; Comox; Laratrim; Septrin	antibacterial
crisantapase	Erwinase	leukaemia
crotamiton	Eurax	antipruritic
cyanocobalamin	Cytacon; Cytamen	anti-anaemic
cyclandelate	Cyclobral; Cyclo-spasmol	vasodilator
cyclizine	Marzine; Valoid	anti-emetic
cyclofenil	Rehibin	infertility
cyclopenthiazide	Navidrex	diuretic
cyclopentolate	Mydrilate	mydriatic
cyclophosphamide	Endoxana	cytotoxic
cyclosporin	Sandimmun	immunosuppressant
cyproheptadine	Periactin	antihistamine
cyproterone	Androcur; Cyprostat	anti-androgen
cytarabine	Alexan; Cytosar	cytotoxic
dacarbazine	DTIC	cytotoxic
danazol	Danol	endometriosis
dantrolene	Dantrium	muscle relaxant
debrisoquine	Declinax	hypertension
demeclocycline	Ledermycin	antibiotic
desferrioxamine	Desferal	iron poisoning
desipramine	Pertofran	antidepressant
desmopressin	DDAVP	diabetes insipidus
desoxymethasone	Stiedex	topical corticosteroid
dexamethasone	Decadron; Oradexon	corticosteroid
dexamphetamine	Dexedrine	appetite suppressant
dexfenfluamine	Adifax	appetite suppressant

Approved Name	Proprietary Name	Main action or Indication
dextran	Gentran; Lomodex; Rheomacrodex	plasma substitute
dextromoramide	Palfium	analgesic
diazepam	Alupram; Atensine; Diazemuls; Stesolid; Valium	tranquillizer
diazoxide	Eudemine	hypertension; hypoglycaemia
dichlorphenamide	Daranide	glaucoma
diclofenac	Rhumalgan; Voltarol	antirheumatic
dicobalt edetate	Kelocyanor	cyanide poisoning
dicyclomine	Merbentyl	antispasmodic
diethylcarbamazine	Banocide	filariasis
diethylpropion	Tenuate	appetite suppressant
diflucortolone	Nerison	topical corticosteroid
diflunisal	Dolobid	analgesic
digoxin	Lanoxin; Lanoxin PG	heart failure
digoxin antibody	Digibind	digoxin overdose
dihydrocodeine	D.F.118	analgesic
dihydroergotamine	Dihydergot	migraine
dihydrotachysterol	A.T.10; Tachyrol	hypocalcaemia
diloxanide furoate	Furamide	amoebiasis
diltiazem	Adizem; Britiazim; Tildiem	calcium antagonist
dimenhydrinate	Dramamine	antihistamine
dimethindene	Fenostil	antihistamine
dinoprost	Prostin F2	uterine stimulant
dinoprostone	Prostin E2	uterine stimulant
diphenoxylate	Lomotil	diarrhoea
diphenylpyraline	Histryl	antihistamine
dipivefrine	Propine	glaucoma
dipyridamole	Persantin	vasodilator
disodium etidronate	Didronel	Paget's disease
disodium pamidronate	Aredia	Paget's disease
disopyramide	Dirythmin-SA; Rythmoden	cardiac arrhythmias
distigmine	Ubretid	urinary retention

Approved Name	**Proprietary Name**	**Main action or Indication**
disulfiram	Antabuse	alcoholism
dithranol triacetate	Exolan	psoriasis
dobutamine	Dobutrex	cardiac stimulant
docusate sodium	Dioctyl	laxative
domperidone	Evoxin; Motilium	anti-emetic
dopamine	Intropin	cardiac stimulant
dopexamine	Dopacard	cardiac surgery
dothiepin	Prothiaden	antidepressant
doxapram	Dopram	respiratory stimulant
doxazosin	Cardura	hypertension
doxepin	Sinequan	antidepressant
doxorubicin	Adriamycin	cytotoxic
doxycycline	Nordox; Vibramycin	antibiotic
droperidol	Droleptan	neuroleptic
dydrogesterone	Duphaston	progestogen
econazole	Ecostatin; Pevaryl	antifungal
ecothiopate iodide	Phospholine iodide	glaucoma
edrophonium	Tensilon	diagnostic
enalapril	Innovace	ACE inhibitor
enflurane	Enthrane	inhalation anaesthetic
enoxacin	Comprecin	antibacterial
enoximone	Perfan	heart failure
enoxaparin	Clexane	thrombosis
epirubicin	Pharmorubicin	cytotoxic
epoetin alpha	Eprex; Recormon	anaemia in chronic renal failure
epoprostenol	Flolan	bypass surgery
ergotamine	Lingraine	migraine
erythromycin	Erythrocin; Ilotycin	antibiotic
esmolol	Brevibloc	beta-blocker
estramustine	Estracyt	cytotoxic
estropipate	Harmogen	oestrogen
ethacrynic acid	Edecrin	diuretic
ethambutol	Myambutol	tuberculosis
ethamivan	Clairvan	respiratory stimulant
ethamsylate	Dicynene	haemostatic
ethoglucid	Epodyl	cytotoxic
ethosuximide	Emeside; Zarontin	anticonvulsant
ethynodiol	Femulen	contraceptive
etidronate	Didronel	Paget's disease
etodolac	Lodine	arthritis
etomidate	Hypnomidate	i.v. anaesthetic

Approved Name	Proprietary Name	Main action or Indication
etoposide	Vepesid	cytotoxic
etretinate	Tigason	psoriasis
Factor VIII	Monoclate-P	haemophilia
famotidine	Pepcid-PM	H_2-blocker
felodipine	Plendil	calcium antagonist
fenbufen	Lederfen	antirheumatic
fenfluramine	Ponderax	appetite suppressant
fenofibrate	Lipantil	hyperlipidaemia
fenoprofen	Fenopron; Progesic	arthritis
fenoterol	Berotec	bronchitis
fentanyl	Sublimaze	analgesic
filgrastim	Neupogen	neutropenia
flavoxate	Urispas	antispasmodic
flecainide	Tambocor	cardiac arrhythmias
fluclorolone	Topilar	topical corticosteroid
flucloxacillin	Floxapen; Ladropen	antibiotic
fluconazole	Diflucan	antifungal
flucytosine	Alcobon	antifungal
fludrocortisone	Florinef	corticosteroid
flumazenil	Anexate	benzodiazepine antagonist
flunisolide	Syntaris	corticosteroid
flunitrazepam	Rohypnol	hypnotic
fluocinolone	Synalar	topical corticosteroid
fluocinonide	Metosyn	topical corticosteroid
fluocortolone	Ultralanum	topical corticosteroid
fluorometholone	FML	topical corticosteroid
fluoxetine	Prozac	antidepressant
flupenthixol	Depixol	schizophrenia
fluphenazine	Modecate; Moditen	schizophrenia
flurandrenolone	Haelan	topical corticosteroid
flurazepam	Dalmane	hypnotic
flurbiprofen	Froben	arthritis
fluspirilene	Redeptin	schizophrenia
fluticasone	Flixonase	topical corticosteroid
flutamide	Drogenil	prostatic carcinoma
fluvoxamine	Faverin	antidepressant
folinic acid	Refolinon	methotrexate antidote
foscarnet	Foscavir	antiviral
fosfestrol	Honvan	cytotoxic
fosfinopril	Staril	ACE inhibitor

Approved Name	Proprietary Name	Main action or Indication
framycetin	Framygen; Soframycin	antibiotic
frusemide	Aluzine; Diuresal; Dryptal; Lasix	diuretic
gallamine	Flaxedil	muscle relaxant
gamolenic acid	Epogam	eczema
ganciclovir	Cymevene	antiviral
gelatin	Gelofusine	blood volume expander
gemeprost	Cervagem	prostaglandin
genfibrozil	Lopid	hyperlipidaemia
gentamicin	Cidomycin; Genticin	antibiotic
gestrinone	Dimetriose	endometriosis
gestronol	Depostat	endometrical carcinoma
glibenclamide	Daonil; Euglucon	hypoglycaemic
gliclazide	Glibenese; Minodiab	hypoglycaemic
gliquidone	Glurenorm	hypoglycaemic
glutaraldehyde	Glutarol	warts
glyceryl trinitrate	Sustac; Tridil	angina
glycopyrronium	Robinul	peptic ulcer
glymidine	Gondafon	hypoglycaemic
gonadorelin	Fertiral	infertility
goserlin	Zoladex	prostatic carcinoma
granisetron	Kytril	migraine
griseofulvin	Fulcin; Grisovin	antifungal
guanethidine	Ismelin	hypertension
halcinonide	Halciderm	topical corticosteroid
halfantrine	Halfan	antimalarial
haloperidol	Haldol; Serenace	schizophrenia
halothane	Fluothane	anaesthetic
hetastarch	Hespan	plasma substitute
hexamine hippurate	Hiprex	urinary antiseptic
HA-1A	Centoxin	bacteraemia
hyaluronidase	Hyalase	enzyme
hydralazine	Apresoline	hypertension
hydrochloro-thiazide	Esidrex; Hydro-saluric	diuretic
hydrocortisone	Corlan; Ef-Cortelan; Hydrocortistab; Hydrocortisyl; Hydrocortone	corticosteroid

Approved Name	Proprietary Name	Main action or Indication
hydroflumethiazide	Hydrenox	diuretic
hydroxocobalamin	Cobalin-H; Neo-Cytamen	anti-anaemic
hydroxychloro-quine	Plaquenil	antimalarial
hydroxy-progesterone	Proluton-Depot	progestogen
hydroxyurea	Hydrea	cytotoxic
hydroxyzine	Atarax	tranquillizer
hyoscine butyl bromide	Buscopan	antispasmodic
ibuprofen	Brufen; Ebufac	arthritis
idarubicin	Zavedos	cytotoxic
idoxuridine	Iduridin; Kerecid	antiviral
ifosfamide	Mitoxana	cytotoxic
imipenem	Primaxin	antibiotic
imipramine	Tofranil	antidepressant
immunoglobulin G	Endobulin	antibody deficiency
indapamide	Natrilix	hypertension
indomethacin	Flexin; Imbrilon; Indocid; Indolar; Indomod; Mobilan; Rheumacin; Slo-Indo	arthritis
indoramin	Baratol	beta-blocker
inosine pranobex	Imunovir	antiviral
inositol nicotinate	Hexopal	vasodilator
interferon	Intron; Roferon; Wellferon	leukaemia
ipratropium	Atrovent	bronchodilator
iprindole	Prondol	antidepressant
iron-dextran	Imferon	iron-deficiency anaemia
iron-sorbitol	Jectofer	iron-deficiency anaemia
isoaminile	Dimyril	antitussive
isocarboxazid	Marplan	antidepressant
isoconazole	Travogyn	candidiasis
isoflurane	Forane	inhalation anaesthetic
isoprenaline	Saventrine	bronchospasm
isosorbide dinitrate	Cedocard; Isoket; Isordil; Sorbitrate; Vascardin	angina

Approved Name	Proprietary Name	Main action or Indication
isosorbide mononitrate	Elantan; Imdur; Ismo; Isotrate; Monit	angina
isotretinoin	Roaccutane	severe acne
isoxuprine	Duvadilan	premature labour
isradipine	Prescal	calcium antagonist
itraconazole	Sporanox	antifungal
ivermectin	Mectizan	filariasis
kanamycin	Kannasyn	antibiotic
ketamine	Ketalar	anaesthetic
ketoconazole	Nizoral	antifungal
ketoprofen	Alrheumat; Orudis	arthritis
ketorolac	Toradol	analgesic
ketotifen	Zaditen	anti-asthmatic
labetalol	Labrocol; Trandate	beta-blocker
lactulose	Duphalac	laxative
lamotrigine	Lamictal	epilepsy
lanatoside C	Cedilanid	cardiac failure
leuprorelin	Prostap	prostatic carcinoma
levobunolol	Betagan	glaucoma
levodopa	Brocadopa; Larodopa	parkinsonism
lignocaine	Xylocaine; Xylocard	anaesthetic
lincomycin	Lincocin	antibiotic
lindane	Quellada	pediculosis
liothyronine	Tertroxin	thyroid deficiency
lisinopril	Carace; Zestril	ACE inhibitor
lithium carbonate	Camcolit; Phasal	mania
lofepramine	Gamanil	antidepressant
lomustine	CCNU	cytotoxic
loperamide	Arret; Imodium	diarrhoea
loratadine	Clarityn	antihistamine
lorazepam	Almazine; Ativan	tranquillizer
loxapine	Loxapac	antipsychotic
lymecycline	Tetralysal	antibiotic
lypressin	Syntopressin	diabetes insipidus
lysuride	Revanil	parkinsonism
malathion	Derbac; Prioderm	parasiticide
maprotiline	Ludiomil	antidepressant
mazindol	Teronac	appetite suppressant
mebendazole	Vermox	anthelmintic
mebeverine	Colofac	antispasmodic

Approved Name	Proprietary Name	Main action or Indication
mebhydrolin	Fabahistin	antihistamine
mecillinam	Selexidin	antibiotic
medazepam	Farlutal; Nobrium	tranquillizer
medroxy-progesterone	Provera	progestogen
mefenamic acid	Ponstan	arthritis
mefloquine	Larium	malaria
mefruside	Baycaron	diuretic
megestrol	Megace	cytotoxic
melphalan	Alkeran	cytotoxic
menadiol	Synkavit	hypoprothrombinaemia
menotrophin	Perganol	hypogonadism
mepenzolate	Cantil	antispasmodic
meprobamate	Equanil	tranquillizer
meptazinol	Meptid	analgesic
mepyramine	Anthisan	topical antihistamine
mequitazine	Primalan	antihistamine
mercaptopurine	Puri-Nethol	cytotoxic
mesalazine	Asacol; Pentasa	ulcerative colitis
mesna	Utomitexan	urotoxicity due to cyclophosphamide
mesterolone	Pro-Viron	androgen
metaraminol	Aramine	hypotension
metformin	Glucophage	hypoglycaemic
methadone	Physeptone	analgesic
methicillin	Celbenin	antibiotic
methixene	Tremonil	parkinsonism
methocarbamol	Robaxin	muscle relaxant
methohexitone	Brietal	anaesthetic
methotrexate	Matrex	cytotoxic
methotrimeprazine	Nozinan	pain in terminal cancer
methoxamine	Vasoxine	vasoconstrictor
methyclothiazide	Enduron	diuretic
methylcellulose	Celevac	laxative
methylcysteine	Visclair	mucolytic
methyldopa	Aldomet; Dopamet	hypertension
methylpheno-barbitone	Prominal	epilepsy
methylprednisolone	Medrone	corticosteroid
methysergide	Deseril	migraine
metirosine	Demser	phaeochromocytoma

Approved Name	Proprietary Name	Main action or Indication
metoclopramide	Maxolon; Metex; Metramid; Parmid; Primperan	anti-emetic
metolazone	Metenix; Xuret	diuretic
metoprolol	Betaloc; Lopressor	beta-blocker
metronidazole	Flagyl; Zadstat	trichomoniasis
metyrapone	Metopirone	resistant oedema
mexenone	Uvistat	sunscreen
mexiletine	Mexitil	cardiac arrhythmias
mezlocillin	Baypen	antibiotic
mianserin	Bolvidon; Norval	antidepressant
miconazole	Dakterin; Dermon-stat	antifungal
midazolam	Hypnovel	i.v. sedative
mifepristone	Mifegyne	antiprogestogen
milrinone	Primacor	severe heart failure
minocycline	Minocin	antibiotic
minoxidil	Loniten	hypertension
misoprostol	Cytotec	peptic ulcer
mitozantrone	Novantrone	cytotoxic
monosulfiram	Tetmosol	scabies
morphine	MST Continus; Sevredol	analgesic
mupirocin	Bactroban	topical antibiotic
nabilone	Cesamet	anti-emetic
nabumetone	Relifex	arthritis
nadolol	Corgard	beta-blocker
nafarelin	Synarel	endometriosis
naftidrofuryl	Praxilene	vasodilator
nalbuphine	Nubain	analgesic
nalidixic acid	Negram	urinary antiseptic
naloxone	Narcan	narcotic antagonist
naltrexone	Nalorex	opioid dependence
nandrolone	Deca-Durabolin; Durabolin	anabolic steroid
naproxen	Laraflex; Naprosyn	arthritis
natamycin	Pimafucin	antibiotic
nedocromil	Tilade	anti-asthmatic
nefopam	Acupan	analgesic
neostigmine	Prostigmin	myasthenia
netilmicin	Netillin	antibiotic
nicardipine	Cardene	calcium antagonist

Approved Name	Proprietary Name	Main action or Indication
niclosamide	Yomesan	anthelmintic
nicofuranose	Bradilan	vasodilator
nicotinyl alcohol	Ronicol	vasodilator
nicoumalone	Sinthrome	anticoagulant
nifedepine	Adalat; Coracten	calcium antagonist
nimodipine	Nimotop	calcium antagonist
nimorazole	Naxogin	trichomoniasis
nitrazepam	Mogadon; Somnite; Surem	hypnotic
nitrofurantoin	Furadantin; Macrodantin	urinary antiseptic
nizatidine	Axid	H_2-blocker
noradrenaline	Levophed	hypotension
norethisterone	Menzol; Primolut N	progestogen
norfloxacin	Utinor	urinary tract infections
	Noroxin	eye infections
nortriptyline	Allegron; Aventyl	antidepressant
noxythiolin	Noxyflex	antiseptic
nystatin	Nystan	antifungal
octreotide	Sandostatin	carcinoid syndrome
ofloxacin	Tarivid	urinary tract infection
olsalazine	Dipentum	ulcerative colitis
omeprazole	Losec	peptic ulcer
ondansetron	Zofran	anti-emetic
orciprenaline	Alupent	bronchospasm
orphenadrine	Biorphen; Disipal	parkinsonism
oxamniquine	Vansil	anthelmintic
oxatomide	Tinset	antihistamine
oxazepam	Oxanid	tranquillizer
oxitropium	Oxivent	bronchodilator
oxpentifylline	Trental	vasodilator
oxprenolol	Trasicor	beta-blocker
oxybutynin	Ditropan	urinary incontinence
oxymetazoline	Afrazine	nasal decongestant
oxymetholone	Anapolon	anabolic steroid
oxypertine	Integrin	tranquillizer
oxyphenbutazone	Tanderil	ocular inflammation
oxytetracycline	Berkmycen; Imperacin; Terramycin; Unimycin	antibiotic
pancuronium	Pavulon	muscle relaxant
papaveretum	Omnopon	analgesic

Approved Name	Proprietary Name	Main action or Indication
paroxetine	Seroxat	antidepressant
pemoline	Volital	cerebral stimulant
penicillamine	Distamine; Pendramine	Wilson's disease
pentaerythritol tetranitrate	Cardiacap; Mycardol	angina
pentamididine	Pentacarinat	leishmaniasis
pentazocine	Fortral	analgesic
pergolide	Celance	parkinsonism
pericyazine	Neulactil	schizophrenia
perindopril	Coversyl	ACE inhibitor
perphenazine	Fentazin	schizophrenia
phenazocine	Narphen	analgesic
phenelzine	Nardil	antidepressant
phenethicillin	Broxil	antibiotic
phenindamine	Thephorin	antihistamine
phenindione	Dindevan	anticoagulant
pheniramine	Daneral	antihistamine
phenoperidone	Operidine	analgesic
phenoxybenzamine	Dibenyline	vasodilator
phenoxymethyl-penicillin	Distaquaine V-K; V-Cil-k	antibiotic
phentermine	Duromine; Ionamin	appetite suppressant
phentolamine	Rogitine	phaeochromocytoma
phenylbutazone	Butazolidin	ankylosing spondylitis
phenytoin	Epanutin	epilepsy
phytomenadione	Konakion	hypoprothrombinaemia
pimozide	Orap	schizophrenia
pindolol	Visken	beta-blocker
pipenzolate	Piptal	antispasmodic
piperacillin	Pipril	antibiotic
piperazine	Antepar	anthelmintic
pipothiazine	Piportil	antipsychotic
pirbuterol	Exirel	bronchodilator
pirenzepine	Gastrozepin	peptic ulcer
pirentanide	Arelix	diuretic
piroxicam	Feldene	antirheumatic
pivampicillin	Pondocillin	antibiotic
pivmecillinam	Selexid	antibiotic
pizotifen	Sanomigran	migraine
plicamycin	Mithracin	malignant hypercalcaemia

Approved Name	Proprietary Name	Main action or Indication
podophyllotoxin	Condyline	penile warts
poldine	Nacton	antispasmodic
polyestradiol	Estradurin	prostatic carcinoma
polygeline	Haemaccel	blood volume expander
polymyxin B	Aerosporin	antibiotic
polythiazide	Nephril	diuretic
pravastatin	Lipostat	hyperlipidaemia
prazosin	Hypovase	hypertension
prednisolone	Deltacortril; Deltastab; Precortisyl; Prednesol	corticosteroid
prednisone	Decortisyl	corticosteroid
prilocaine	Citanest	anaesthetic
primidone	Mysoline	epilepsy
probenecid	Benemid	gout
probucol	Lurselle	hyperlipidaemia
procainamide	Pronestyl	cardiac arrhythmias
procaine-penicillin	Depocillin	antibiotic
procarbazine	Natulan	cytotoxic
prochlorperazine	Stemetil; Vertigon	anti-emetic; vertigo
procyclidine	Kemadrin	parkinsonism
proguanil	Paludrine	antimalarial
promazine	Sparine	tranquillizer
promethazine	Phenergan	antihistamine
promethazine theoclate	Avomine	anti-emetic
propafenone	Arythmol	cardiac arrhythmias
propamidine	Brolene	conjunctivitis
propantheline	Pro-Banthine	peptic ulcer
propofol	Diprivan	anaesthetic
propranolol	Bedranol; Inderal; Sloprolol	beta-blocker
protriptyline	Concordin	antidepressant
proxymetacaine	Ophthaine	corneal anaesthetic
pyrantel	Combantrin	anthelminitic
pyrazinamide	Zinamide	tuberculosis
pyridostigmine	Nestinon	myasthenia
pyridoxine	Benadon	vitamin B deficiency
pyrimethamine	Daraprim	antimalarial
quinalbarbitone	Seconal	hypnotic
quinapril	Accupro	ACE inhibitor
ramipril	Tritace	ACE inhibitor
ranitidine	Zantac	H_2-blocker

Approved Name	Proprietary Name	Main action or Indication
razoxane	Razoxin	cytotoxic
remoxipride	Roxiam	schizophrenia
reproterol	Bronchodil	bronchodilator
reserpine	Serpasil	hypertension
rifampicin	Rifadin; Rimactane	tuberculosis
rimiterol	Pulmadil	bronchodilator
ritodrine	Yutopar	premature labour
salbutamol	Ventolin	bronchospasm
salcatonin	Calsynar; Miacalcic	Paget's disease
salmeterol	Serevent	bronchospasm
salsalate	Disalcid	antirheumatic
selegiline	Eldepryl	parkinsonism
silver sulphadiazine	Flamazine	antibacterial
simvastatin	Zocor	hyperlipidaemia
sodium aurothiomalate	Myocrisin	rheumatoid arthritis
sodium clodronate	Loron; Bonefos	hypercalcaemia of malignancy
sodium cromoglycate	Intal; Rynacrom	anti-allergic
sodium fusidate	Fucidin	antibiotic
sodium iron edetate	Sytron	anti-anaemia
sodium nitroprusside	Nipride	hypertensive crisis
sodium pico-sulphate	Laxoberal	laxative
sodium stibo-gluconate	Pentostam	leishmaniasis
sodium valproate	Epilim	epilepsy
sotalol	Beta-Cardone; Sotacor	beta-blocker
spectinomycin	Trobicin	antibiotic
spironolactone	Aldactone; Spiroctan	diuretic
stanozolol	Stromba	anabolic steroid
streptokinase	Kabikinase; Streptase	fibrinolytic
sucralfate	Antepsin	peptic ulcer
sulconazole	Exelderm	antifungal
sulfadoxine	Fanosil	antimalarial
sulfametopyrazine	Kelfizine	sulphonamide
sulindac	Clinoril	arthritis
sulphacetamide	Albucid; Ocusol	sulphonamide

Approved Name	Proprietary Name	Main action or Indication
sulphadimidine	Sulphamezathine	sulphonamide
sulphasalazine	Salazopyrin	ulcerative colitis
sulphinpyrazone	Anturan	gout
sultamicin	Unasyn	antibiotic
sumatriptan	Imigran	migraine
suxamethonium	Anectine; Scoline	muscle relaxant
talampicillin	Talpen	antibiotic
tamoxifen	Nolvadex	cytotoxic
teicoplanin	Targocid	antibiotic
temafloxacin	Teflox	antibacterial
temocillin	Temopen	antibiotic
temazepam	Normison	hypnotic
tenoxicam	Mobiflex	arthritis
terazosin	Hytrin	hypertension
terbinafine	Lamisil	antifungal
terbutaline	Bricanyl	bronchospasm
terfenadine	Seldane; Triludan	antihistamine
terolidin	Micturin	urinary frquency
testosterone	Virormone	hypogonadism
tetrabenazine	Nitoman	chorea
tetracosactrin	Synacthen	corticotrophin
tetracycline	Panmycin; Sustamycin; Tetrabid; Tetrachel; Tetrex	antibiotic
theophylline	Biophylline	bronchodilator
thiabendazole	Mintezol	anthelmintic
thiambutosine	Ciba 1906	anthelmintic
thiamine	Benerva	vitamin B_1 deficiency
thiethylperazine	Torecan	anti-emetic
thioguanine	Lanvin	cytotoxic
thiopentone	Intravel	i.v. anaesthetic
thioridazine	Melleril	tranquillizer
thymoxamine	Opilon	vasodilator
thyroxine	Eltroxin	thyroid deficiency
tiaprofenic acid	Surgam	antirheumatic
tibolone	Livial	menopause
ticarcillin	Ticar	antibiotic
timolol	Betim; Blocadren	beta-blocker
tinidazole	Fasigyn	anaerobic infections
tioconazole	Trosyl	antifungal
tocainide	Tonocard	cardiac arrhythmias
tolazamide	Tolanase	hypoglycaemic

Approved Name	Proprietary Name	Main action or Indication
tolbutamide	Rastinon	hypoglycaemic
tolmetin	Tolectin	antirheumatic
tranexamic acid	Cyklokapron	antifibrinolytic
tranylcypromine	Parnate	antidepressant
trazodone	Molipaxin	antidepressant
tretinoin	Retin-A	acne
triamcinolone	Adcortyl; Ledercort	corticosteroid
triamterene	Dytac	diuretic
triazolam	Halcion	hypnotic
tribavirin	Virazid	antiviral
trifluoperazine	Stelazine	tranquillizer
trifluperidol	Triperidol	neuroleptic
trilostane	Modrenal	aldosteronism
trimeprazine	Vallergan	antihistamine
trimetaphan	Arfonad	hypotensive surgery
trimethoprim	Ipral; Monotrim; Syraprim; Trimogal; Trimopan	antibacterial
trimipramine	Surmontil	antidepressant
triprolidine	Actidil	antihistamine
tropicamide	Mydriacyl	mydriatic
tubocurarine	Tubarine	muscle relaxant
tulobuterol	Brelomax	bronchodilator
urokinase	Ukidan	hyphaemia; embolism
ursodeoxycholic acid	Destolit	gallstones
vancomycin	Vancocin	antibiotic
vecuronium	Norcuron	muscle relaxant
verapamil	Cordilox; Univer	angina; hypertension
vidarabine	Vira-A	cytotoxic
vigabatrin	Sabril	anticonvulsant
viloxazine	Vivalan	antidepressant
vinblastine	Velbe	cytotoxic
vincristine	Oncovin	cytotoxic
vindesine	Eldisine	cytotoxic
warfarin	Marevan	anticoagulant
xamoterol	Corwin	mild heart failure
xipamide	Diurexan	diuretic
xylometazoline	Otrivine	nasal decongestant
zidovudine	Retrovir	antiviral (AIDS)
zopiclone	Zimovane	hypnotic
zuclopenthixol	Clopixol	schizophrenia

Proprietary Name	Approved Name	Main action or Indication
Accupro	quinapril	ACE inhibitor
Acepril	captopril	ACE inhibitor
Acetoxyl	benzoyl peroxide	acne
Achromycin	tetracycline	antibiotic
Acthar	corticotropin	hormone
Aclacin	aclarubicin	cytotoxic
Actidil	triprolidine	antihistamine
Actilyse	alteplase	fibrinolytic
Acupan	nefopam	analgesic
Adalat	nifedepine	calcium antagonist
Adcortyl	triamcinolone	topical corticosteroid
Adenocor	adenosine	paroxysmal tachycardia
Adifax	dexfenfluramine	appetite suppressant
Adizem	diltiazem	angina
Adriamycin	doxorubicin	antibiotic
Aerosporin	polymyxin B	antibiotic
Afrazine	oxymetazoline	nasal decongestant
Akineton	biperiden	parkinsonism
Alcobon	flucytosine	antifungal
Alcopar	bephenium	anthelmintic
Aldactide	co-flumactone	diuretic
Aldactone	spironolactone	resistant oedema
Aldomet	methyldopa	hypertension
Alexan	cytarabine	cytotoxic
Alimix	cisapride	oesophageal reflux
Alkeran	melphalan	cytotoxic
Allegron	nortriptyline	antidepressant
Aller-eeze	clemastine	antihistamine
Alloferin	alcuronium	muscle relaxant
Almazine	lorazepam	tranquillizer
Almodan	amoxycillin	antibiotic
Aloral	allopurinol	gout
Alphodith	dithranol	psoriasis
Alrheumet	ketoprofen	arthritis
Aluline	allopurinol	gout
Alumex	chlorpheniramine	antihistamine
Alupent	orciprenaline	bronchodilator
Alupram	diazepam	anxiolytic
Aluzine	frusemide	diuretic
Ambaxin	bacampicillin	antibiotic
Ambilhar	niridizole	anthelmintic
Amfipen	ampicillin	antibiotic

Proprietary Name	Approved Name	Main action or Indication
Amikin	amikacin	antibiotic
Amilco	co-amilozide	diuretic
Amoxil	amoxycillin	antibiotic
Amsidine	amacrine	cytotoxic
Amytal	amylobarbitone	hypnotic
Anaflex	polynoxylin	antiseptic
Anafranil	clomipramine	antidepressant
Anapolon	oxymetholone	anabolic steroid
Androcur	cyproterone	anti-androgen
Anectine	suxamethonium	muscle relaxant
Anexate	flumazenil	benzodiazepine antagonist
Angilol	propranolol	beta-blocker
Angiozem	diltiazem	angina
Anquil	benperidol	tranquillizer
Antabuse	disulfiram	alcoholism
Antepar	piperazine	anthelmintic
Antepsin	sulcralfate	peptic ulcer
Anthisan	mepyramine	topical antihistamine
Anthranol	dithranol	psoriasis
Antraderm	dithranol	psoriasis
Anturan	sulphinpyrazone	gout
Apresoline	hydralazine	hypertension
Aprinox	bendrofluazide	diuretic
Apsifen	ibuprofen	arthritis
Aquadrate	urea	ichthyosis
Aramine	metaraminol	vasoconstrictor
Aredia	disodium pamidronate	hypercalcaemia of malignancy
Arelix	piretanide	hypertension
Arfonad	trimetaphan	hypotensive surgery
Arpicolin	procyclidine	parkinsonism
Arpimycin	erythromycin	antibiotic
Arret	loperamide	diarrhoea
Artane	benzhexol	parkinsonism
Arythmol	propafenone	cardiac arrhythmias
Asacol	mesalazine	ulcerative colitis
Ascabiol	benzyl benzoate	scabies
Asendis	amoxapine	antidepressant
A.T.10	dihydrotachysterol	hypocalcaemia
Atarax	hydroxyzine	tranquillizer
Atensine	diazepam	tranquillizer
Ativan	lorazepam	tranquillizer

Proprietary Name	Approved Name	Main action or Indication
Atromid-S	clofibrate	hypercholesterolaemia
Atrovent	ipratropium	bronchodilator
Aureomycin	chlortetracycline	antibiotic
Augmentin	co-amoxiclav	antibiotic
Aventyl	nortriptyline	antidepressant
Avoclor	chloroquine	antimalarial
Avomine	promethazine theoclate	anti-emetic
Axid	nizatidine	H_2-blocker
Azactam	aztreonam	antibiotic
Azamune	azathioprine	cytotoxic
Bactrim	co-trimoxazole	antibacterial
Bactroban	mupirocin	topical antibiotic
Banocide	diethylcarbamazine	filariasis
Baratol	indoramin	beta-blocker
Baxan	cefadroxil	antibiotic
Baycaron	mefruside	diuretic
Baypen	mezlocillin	antibiotic
Becloforte	beclomethasone	corticosteroid
Beconase	beclomethasone	rhinitis
Becotide	beclomethasone	corticosteroid
Bedranol SR	propranolol	beta-blocker
Benadon	pyridoxine	vitamin B_6 deficiency
Bendogen	bethanidine	hypertension
Benemid	probenecid	gout
Benerva	thiamine	vitamin B_1 deficiency
Benoral	benorylate	analgesic
Benoxyl	benzyl peroxide	acne
Bentex	benzhexol	parkinsonism
Benzagel	benzyl peroxide	acne
Berkaprine	azathioprine	cytotoxic
Berkatens	verapamil	angina; hypertension
Berkmycen	oxytetracycline	antibiotic
Berkolol	propranolol	beta-blocker
Berkozide	bendrofluazide	diuretic
Berotec	fenoterol	bronchitis
Beta-Cardone	sotalol	beta-blocker
Betadine	povidone-iodine	antiseptic
Betadren	pindolol	beta-blocker
Betagan	levobunolol	glaucoma
Betaloc	metoprolol	beta-blocker
Betim	timolol	beta-blocker
Betnelan	betamethasone	corticosteroid

Proprietary Name	Approved Name	Main action or Indication
Betnesol	betamethasone	corticosteroid
Betnovate	betamethasone	topical corticosteroid
Betoptic	betaxolol	glaucoma
Bezalip	bezafibrate	hyperlipidaemia
BiCNU	carmustine	cytotoxic
Biltricide	praziquantel	anthelmintic
Biogastrone	carbenoxolone	peptic ulcer
Biophylline	theophylline	bronchodilator
Bioplex	carbenoxolone	oral ulcers
Biorphen	orphenadrine	parkinsonism
Blocadren	timolol	beta-blocker
Bolvidon	mianserin	antidepressant
Bonefos	sodium clodronate	hypercalcaemia of malignancy
Bradilan	nicofuranose	vasodilator
Brelomax	tulobuterol	bronchodilator
Bretylate	bretylium	cardiac arrhythmias
Brevibloc	esmolol	beta-blocker
Bricanyl	terbutaline	bronchospasm
Brietal	methohexitone	anaesthetic
Britiazim	diltiazem	angina
Brocadopa	levodopa	parkinsonism
Broflex	benzhexol	parkinsonism
Brolene	propamidine	conjunctivitis
Bronchodil	reproterol	bronchodilator
Brufen	ibuprofen	arthritis
Buccastem	prochlorperazine	vertigo
Burinex	bumetanide	diuretic
Buscopan	hyoscine butyl bromide	antispasmodic
Buspar	buspirone	anxiolytic
Butazolidin	phenylbutazone	ankylosing spondylitis
Cacit	calcium carbonate	osteoporosis
Calabren	glibenclamide	hypoglycaemic
Calciparine	calcium heparin	anticoagulant
Calcisorb	sodium cellulose phosphate	hypercalciuria
Calcitare	calcitonin	Paget's disease
Calcium Resonium	exchange resin	hyperkalaemia
Calpol	paracetamol	analgesic
Calsynar	salcatonin	Paget's disease
Camcolit	lithium carbonate	mania
Canestan	clotrimazole	antifungal

Proprietary Name	Approved Name	Main action or Indication
Cantil	mepenzolate	antispasmodic
Capastat	capreomycin	tuberculosis
Caplenal	allopurinol	gout
Capoten	captopril	ACE inhibitor
Caprin	aspirin	arthritis
Carace	lisinopril	ACE inhibitor
Cardene	nicardipine	angina
Cardiacap	pentaerythritol	angina
Cardinol	propranolol	beta-blocker
Cardura	doxazosin	hypertension
Carisoma	carisprodol	muscle relaxant
Cartrol	carteolol	beta-blocker
Carylderm	carbaryl	parasiticide
Catapres	clonidine	hypertension
CCNU	lomustine	cytotoxic
Cedilanid	lanatoside C	heart failure
Cedocard	isosorbide dinitrate	angina
Cefizox	ceftizoxime	antibiotic
Celance	pergolide	parkinsonism
Celbenin	methicillin	antibiotic
Celectol	celiprolol	hypertension
Celevac	methylcellulose	laxative
Centoxin	HA-1A	bacteraemia
Centyl	bendrofluazide	diuretic
Ceporex	cephalexin	antibiotic
Cervagem	gemeprost	prostaglandin
Cesamet	nabilone	anti-emetic
Cetavlex	cetrimide	antiseptic
Chendol	chenodeoxycholic acid	gallstones
Chenofalk	chenodeoxycholic acid	gallstones
Chloromycetin	chloramphenicol	antibiotic
Choledyl	choline theophyllinate	bronchodilator
Ciba 1906	thiambutosine	leprosy
Cidomycin	gentamicin	antibiotic
Cinobac	cinoxacin	antibiotic
Ciproxin	ciprofloxacin	antibacterial
Citanest	prilocaine	anaesthetic
Claforan	cefotaxime	antibiotic
Clairvan	ethamivan	respiratory stimulant
Clarityn	loratadine	antihistamine

Proprietary Name	Approved Name	Main action or Indication
Clexane	enoxaparin	thrombosis
Clinoril	sulindac	arthritis
Clomid	clomiphene	gonadotrophin inhibitor
Clopixol	zuclopenthixol	schizophrenia
Clozaril	clozapine	antipsychotic
Cobalin H	hydroxocobalamin	anti-anaemic
Codis	co-codamol	analgesic
Cogentin	benztropine	parkinsonism
Colestid	colestipol	exchange resin
Colofac	mebeverine	antispasmodic
Colomycin	colistin	antibiotic
Colpermin	peppermint oil	antispasmodic
Combantrin	pyrantel	anthelmintic
Comox	co-trimoxazole	antibacterial
Comprecin	enoxacin	antibacterial
Concordin	protriptyline	antidepressant
Condyline	podophyllotoxin	penile warts
Coparvax	vaccine	immunostimulant
Coracten	nifedipine	calcium antagonist
Cordarone X	amiodarone	cardiac arrhythmias
Cordilox	verapamil	angina
Corgard	nadolol	beta-blocker
Corlan	hydrocortisone	local corticosteroid
Coro-Nitro	glyceryl trinitrate	angina
Corsodyl	chlorhexidine	antiseptic
Cortelan	cortisone	corticosteroid
Cortistab	cortisone	corticosteroid
Cortisyl	cortisone	corticosteroid
Corwin	xamoterol	mild heart failure
Cosmegen	actinomycin D	cytotoxic
Coversyl	perindopril	ACE inhibitor
Creon	pancreatin	cystic fibrosis
Crystapen	benzylpenicillin	antibiotic
Cyclobral	cyclandelate	vasodilator
Cyclogest	progesterone	pre-menstrual syndrome
Cyclospasmol	cyclandelate	vasodilator
Cyklokapron	tranexamic acid	antifibrinolytic
Cymevene	ganciclovir	antiviral
Cyprostat	cyproterone	prostatic carcinoma
Cytacon	cyanocobalamin	anti-anaemic
Cytamen	cyanocobalamin	anti-anaemic
Cytosar	cytarabine	cytotoxic
Cytotec	misoprostol	peptic ulcer

Proprietary Name	Approved Name	Main action or Indication
Daktarin	miconazole	antifungal
Dalacin C	clindamycin	antibiotic
Dalmane	flurazepam	hypnotic
Daneral SA	pheniramine	antihistamine
Danol	danazol	endometriosis
Dantrium	dantrolene	muscle relaxant
Daonil	glibenclamide	hypoglycaemic
Daranide	dichlorphenamide	glaucoma
Daraprim	pyrimethamine	antimalarial
DDAVP	desmopressin	diabetes insipidus
Decadron	dexamethasone	corticosteroid
Deca-Durabolin	nandrolone	cytotoxic
Declinax	debrisoquine	hypertension
Decortisyl	prednisone	corticosteroid
Deltacortril	prednisolone	corticosteroid
Deltastab	prednisolone	corticosteroid
Demser	metirosine	phaeochromocytoma
De-Nol	bismuth chelate	peptic ulcer
Depixol	flupenthixol	schizophrenia
Deponit	glyceryl trinitratre	angina
Depostat	gestronol	endometrial carcinoma
Derbac	carbaryl	parasiticide
Dermovate	clobetasol	topical corticosteroid
Deseril	methysergide	migraine
Desferal	desferrioxamine	iron poisoning
Destolit	ursodeoxycholic acid	gallstones
Dexedrine	dexamphetamine	appetite depressant
Dextraven 110	dextran	plasma substitute
D.F.118	dihydrocodeine	analgesic
Diabinese	chlorpropamide	hypoglycaemic
Diamicron	glicazide	hypoglycaemic
Diamox	acetazolamide	glaucoma
Diatensec	spironolactone	congestive heart failure
Diazemuls	diazepam	anxiolytic
Dibenyline	phenoxybenzamine	vasodilator
Dicynene	ethamsylate	haemostatic
Didronel	disodium etidronate	Paget's disease
Diflucan	fluconazole	antifungal
Digibind	digoxin antibody	digoxin overdose
Dihydergot	dehydroergotamine	migraine
Dimetriose	gestrinone	endometriosis

Proprietary Name	Approved Name	Main action or Indication
Dimotane	brompheniramine	antihistamine
Dimyril	isoaminile	antitussive
Dindevan	phenindione	anticoagulant
Dioctyl	docusate sodium	laxative
Dipentum	olsalazine	ulcerative colitis
Diprivan	propofol	IV anaesthetic
Dirythmin-SA	disopyramide	cardiac arrhythmias
Disalcid	salsalate	antirheumatic
Disipal	orphenadrine	parkinsonism
Distaclor	cefaclor	antibiotic
Distamine	penicillamine	Wilson's disease
Distaquaine V-K	phenoxymethyl penicillin	antibiotic
Ditropan	oxybutynin	urinary incontinence
Diuresal	frusemide	diuretic
Diurexan	xipamide	diuretic
Dixarit	clonidine	migraine
Dobutrex	dobutamine	cardiac stimulant
Dolmatil	sulpiride	schizophrenia
Dolobid	diflunisal	analgesic
Doloxene	dextropropoxy-phene	analgesic
Domical	amitriptyline	antidepressant
Dopacard	dopexamine	cardiac surgery
Dopamet	methyldopa	hypertension
Dopram	doxopram	respiratory stimulant
Doralase	indoramin	hypertension
Dovonex	calcipotriol	psoriasis
Dozic	haloperidol	antipsychotic
Dramamine	dimenhydrinate	antihistamine
Drogenil	flutamide	prostatic carcinoma
Droleptan	droperidol	analgesic
Dryptal	frusemide	diuretic
DTIC	dacarbazine	cytotoxic
Dulcolax	bisacodyl	laxative
Duphalac	lactulose	laxative
Duphaston	dydrogestone	progestogen
Durabolin	nandrolone	anabolic steroid
Duromine	phentermine	appetite suppressant
Duvadilan	isoxuprine	vasodilator
Dyspamet	cimetidine	H_2-blocker
Dysport	botulinum toxin	blepharospasm
Dytac	triamterine	diuretic

Proprietary Name	Approved Name	Main action or Indication
Ebufac	ibuprofen	arthritis
Ecostatin	econazole	antifungal
Edecrin	ethacrynic acid	diuretic
Efalith	lithium succinate	seborrhoea
Ef-Cortelan	hydrocortisone	topical corticosteroid
Efudix	fluorouracil	cytotoxic
Elantan	isosorbide mononitrate	angina
Eldepryl	selegiline	parkinsonism
Eldisine	vindesine	cytotoxic
Eltroxin	thyroxine	thyroid defeciency
Elyzol	metronidazole	anaerobic infections
Emblon	tamoxifen	cytotoxic
Emcor	bisoprolol	beta-blocker
Emeside	ethosuximide	anticonvulsant
Emflex	acemetacin	arthritis
Eminase	anistreplase	fibrinolytic
Endobulin	immunoglobulin G	antibody deficiency
Endoxana	cyclophosphamide	cytotoxic
Enduron	methyclothiazide	diuretic
Epanutin	phenytoin	anticonvulsant
Ephynal	tocopherol	vitamin E deficiency
Epifrin	adrenaline	glaucoma
Epilim	sodium valproate	anticonvulsant
Epogam	gamolenic acid	eczema
Eppy	adrenaline	glaucoma
Eprex	erythropoietin	anaemia in chronic renal failure
Equanil	meprobamate	tranquillizer
Eradacin	acrosoxacin	gonorrhoea
Erwinase	crisantaspase	leukaemia
Erycen	erythromycin	antibiotic
Erymax	erythromycin	antibiotic
Erythrocin	erythromycin	antibiotic
Erythromin	erythromycin	antibiotic
Erythroped	erythromycin	antibiotic
Esbatal	bethanidine	hypertension
Esidrex	hydrochlorothiazide	diuretic
Estracyt	estramustine	cytotoxic
Estradurin	polyestradiol	prostatic carcinoma
Eudemine	diazoxide	hypertension; hypoglycaemia

Proprietary Name	Approved Name	Main action or Indication
Euglucon	glibenclamide	hypoglycaemic
Eumovate	clobetasone	topical corticosteroid
Eurax	crotamiton	antipruritic
Evadyne	butriptyline	antidepressant
Evoxin	domperidone	anti-emetic
Exirel	pirbuterol	bronchodilator
Exolan	dithranol triacetate	psoriasis
Exosurf	colfosceril	neonatal respiratory distress
Fabahistin	mebhydrolin	antihistamine
Fabrol	acetylcysteine	mucolytic
Farlutal	medroxy-progesterone	progestogen
Fasigyn	tinidazole	anaerobic infections
Faverin	fluvoxamine	antidepressant
Feldene	piroxicam	arthritis
Femulen	ethynodiol	oral contraceptive
Fenbid	ibuprofen	arthritis
Fenopron	fenoprofen	arthritis
Fenostil	dimethindene	antihistamine
Fentazin	perphenazine	tranquillizer
Fertiral	gonadorelin	infertility
Flagyl	metronidazole	trichomoniasis
Flamazine	silver sulphadiazine	antibacterial
Flaxedil	gallamine	muscle relaxant
Flixonase	fluticasone	topical corticosteroid
Flolan	epoprostenol	preserving platelet function in by-pass surgery
Florinef	fludrocortisone	corticosteroid
Floxapen	flucloxacillin	antibiotic
Flu-Amp	co-fluampicil	antibiotic
Fluanoxol	flupenthixol	antidepressant
Fluothane	halothane	inhalation anaesthetic
FML	fluoromethalone	topical corticosteroid
Forane	isoflurane	inhalation anaesthetic
Fortral	pentazocine	analgesic
Fortum	ceftazidime	antibiotic
Fortunan	haloperidol	antipsychotic
Foscavir	foscarnet	antiviral
Fragmin	heparin	anticoagulant
Framygen	framycetin	antibiotic
Frisium	clobazam	anxiolytic
Froben	flurbiprofen	antirheumatic

Proprietary Name	Approved Name	Main action or Indication
Frumil	co-amilofruse	diuretic
Fucidin	sodium fusidate	antibiotic
Fulcin	griseofulvin	antifungal
Fungilin	amphotericin B	antifungal
Fungizone	amphotericin B	antifungal
Furadantin	nitrofurantoin	urinary antiseptic
Furamide	diloxanide furoate	amoebiasis
Galcodine	codeine	antitussive
Galenphol	pholcodine	antitussive
Galenamox	amoxycillin	antibiotic
Gamanil	lofepramine	antidepressant
Garamycin	gentamicin	antibiotic
Gastromax	metoclopramide	anti-emetic
Gastrozepin	pirenzepine	peptic ulcer
Gelofusin	gelatin	blood volume expander
Genotropin	somatropin	growth hormone
Genticin	gentamicin	antibiotic
Gentran	dextran	plasma substitute
Gestanin	allyloestranol	progestogen
Glibenese	glipizide	hypoglycaemic
Glucophage	metformin	hypoglycaemic
Glucotard	guar gum	hypoglycaemic
Glurenorm	gliquidone	hypoglycaemic
Glypressin	terlipressin	oesophageal varices
Grisovin	griseofulvin	antifungal
Guarem	guar gum	hypoglycaemic
Haelan	fluandrenolone	topical corticosteroid
Halciderm	halcinonide	topical corticosteroid
Halcion	triazolam	hypnotic
Haldol	haloperidol	schizophrenia
Halfan	halofantrine	antimalarial
Hamarin	allopurinol	gout
Harmogen	oestrone	menopause
Heminevrin	chlormethiazole	psychosis; hypnotic
Hep-Flush	heparin	anticoagulant
Heplok	heparin	anticoagulant
Hepsal	heparin	anticoagulant
Herpid	idoxuridine	antiviral
Hespan	hetastarch	plasma substitute
Hexopal	inositol nicotinate	vasodilator
Hibitane	chlorhexidine	antiseptic
Hiprex	hexamine hippurate	urinary antiseptic
Hismanal	astemizole	antihistamine

Proprietary Name	Approved Name	Main action or Indication
Histryl	diphenylpyraline	antihistamine
Honvan	fosfestrol	cytotoxic
Humatrope	somatropin	growth hormone
Humegon	gonadotrophin	infertility
Hyalase	hyaluronidase	enzyme
Hydergine	co-dergocrine	dementia
Hydrea	hydroxyurea	cytotoxic
Hydrenox	hydroflumethiazide	diuretic
Hydrocortistab	hydrocortisone	corticosteroid
Hydrocortisyl	hydrocortisone	corticosteroid
Hydrocortone	hydrocortisone	corticosteroid
Hydrosaluric	hydrochloro-thiazide	diuretic
Hygroton	chlorthalidone	diuretic
Hypertane 50	co-amilozide	diuretic
Hypnomidate	etomidate	IV anaesthetic
Hypnovel	midazolam	hypnotic
Hypovase	prazosin	hypertension
Hytrin	terazocin	hypertension
Ibular	ibuprofen	arthritis
Idoxene	idoxuridine	antiviral
Iduridin	idoxuridine	antiviral
Ilosone	erythromycin	antibiotic
Imbrilon	indomethacin	arthritis
Imdur	isosorbide mono-nitrate	angina
Imferon	iron-dextran	iron-deficiency anaemia
Imigran	sumatriptan	migraine
Immunoprin	azathioprine	immunosuppressant
Imodium	loperamide	diarrhoea
Imperacin	oxytetracycline	antibiotic
Imunovir	inosine pranobex	antiviral
Imuran	azathioprine	immunosuppressant
Inderal	propranolol	beta-blocker
Indocid	indomethacin	arthritis
Indolar SR	indomethacin	arthritis
Indomod	indomethacin	arthritis
Innovace	enalapril	ACE inhibitor
Inoven	ibuprofen	analgesic
Intal	sodium cromoglycate	asthma
Integrin	oxypertine	antipsychotic
Intraval	thiopentone	IV anaesthetic

Proprietary Name	Approved Name	Main action or Indication
Intron A	interferon	leukaemia
Intropin	dopamine	cardiac stimulant
Iodosorb	cadexomer iodine	leg ulcers
Ionamin	phentamine	appetite suppressant
Ipral	trimethoprim	antibacterial
Ismelin	guanethidine	hypertension
Ismo	isosorbide mononitrate	angina
Isordil	isosorbide dinitrate	angina
Isotrate	isosorbide mononitrate	angina
Istin	amlodipine	calcium antagonist
Jectofer	iron-sorbitol	iron deficiency anaemia
Jexin	tubocurarine	muscle relaxant
Kabikinase	streptokinase	fibrinolytic
Kannasyn	kanamycin	antibiotic
Kefadol	cefamandole	antibiotic
Keflex	cephalexin	antibiotic
Keflin	cephalothin	antibiotic
Kefzol	cephazolin	antibiotic
Kelfizine	sulfametopyrazine	sulphonamide
Kelocyanor	dicobalt edetate	cyanide poisoning
Kemadrin	procyclidine	parkinsonism
Kemicetine	chloromycetin	antibiotic
Kenalog	triamcinolone	corticosteroid
Kerecid	idoxuridine	antiviral
Kerlone	betaxolol	beta-blocker
Ketalar	ketamine	IV anaesthetic
Kiditard	quinidine	cardiac arrhythmias
Kinidin	quinidine	cardiac arrhythmias
Klaricid	clarithromycin	antibiotic
Konakion	phytomenadione	hypoprothrombinaemia
Kytril	granisetron	anti-emetic
Labrocol	labetalol	beta-blocker
Ladropen	flucloxacillin	antibiotic
Lamictal	lamotrigine	epilepsy
Lamisil	terbinafine	antifungal agent
Lamprene	clofazimine	leprosy
Lanoxin	digoxin	heart failure
Lanvis	thioguanine	cytotoxic
Laractone	spironolactone	diuretic
Laraflex	naproxen	arthritis
Larapam	piroxicam	arthritis

Proprietary Name	Approved Name	Main action or Indication
Laratrim	co-trimoxazole	antibacterial
Largactil	chlorpromazine	antipsychotic
Larium	mefloquine	malaria
Larodopa	levodopa	parkinsonism
Lasix	frusemide	diuretic
Lasma	theophylline	bronchodilator
Lasoride	co-amilofruse	diuretic
Laxoberal	sodium picosulphate	laxative
Ledercort	triamcinolone	corticosteroid
Lederfen	fenbufen	antirheumatic
Ledermycin	demeclocycline	antibiotic
Lederspan	triamcinolone	corticosteriod
Lentizol	amitriptyline	antidepressant
Leukeran	chlorambucil	cytotoxic
Levophed	noradrenaline	vasoconstrictor
Lexotan	bromazepam	anxiolytic
Libanil	glibenclamide	hypoglycaemic
Librium	chlordiazepoxide	antipsychotic
Lidifen	ibuprofen	arthritis
Limclair	trisodium edetate	ocular lime burns
Lincocin	lincomycin	antibiotic
Lingraine	ergotamine	migraine
Lioresal	baclofen	muscle relaxant
Lipantil	fenofibrate	hyperlipidaemia
Lipostat	pravastatin	hyperlipidaemia
Liskonum	lithium carbonate	mania
Litarex	lithium citrate	mania
Livial	tibolone	menopausal symptoms
Loceryl	amorolfine	topical antifungal
Lodine	etodolac	arthritis
Lomodex	dextran	plasma substitute
Lomotil	co-phenotrope	diarrhoea
Loniten	minoxidil	hypertension
Lopid	gemfibrozil	hyperlipidaemia
Lopressor	metoprolol	beta-blocker
Loron	sodium clodronate	hypercalcaemia of malignancy
Losec	omeprazole	peptic ulcer
Loxapac	loxapine	antipsychotic
Ludiomil	maprotiline	antidepressant
Lurselle	probucol	hyperlipidaemia
Macrodantin	nitrofurantoin	urinary infections

Proprietary Name	Approved Name	Main action or Indication
Macrodox	dextran	plasma substitute
Madopar	co-beneldopa	parkinsonism
Magnapen	co-fluampicil	antibiotic
Malinal	almasilate	antacid
Mantadine	amantadine	parkinsonism
Marcain	bupivacaine	anaesthetic
Marevan	warfarin	anticoagulant
Marplan	isocarboxazid	antidepressant
Maxolon	metoclopramide	anti-emetic
Maxtrex	methotrexate	cytotoxic
Marzine	cinnarizine	anti-emetic
Mectizan	ivermectin	filariasis
Medocodone	co-codamol	analgesic
Medrone	methylprednisolone	corticosteroid
Mefoxin	cefoxitin	antibiotic
Megace	megestrol	cytotoxic
Megaclor	clomocycline	antibiotic
Melleril	thioridazine	tranquillizer
Menzol	norethhisterone	menorrhagia
Meptid	meptazinol	analgesic
Merbentyl	dicyclomine	antispasmodic
Mestinon	pyridostigmine	myasthenia
Metenix	metolazone	diuretic
Metopirone	metyrapone	resistant oedema
Metosyn	fluocinonide	corticosteroid
Metox	metoclopramide	anti-emetic
Metramid	metoclopramide	anti-emetic
Metrodin	urofollitrophin	infertility
Metrolyl	metronidazole	amoebicide
Mexitil	mexilitene	cardiac arrhythmias
Miacalcic	salcatonin	Paget's disease
Micturin	terolidine	urinary frequency
Midamor	amiloride	diuretic
Mifegyne	mifepristone	antiprogestogen
Minocin	minocycline	antibiotic
Minodiab	glipizide	hypoglycaemic
Mintec	peppermint oil	antispasmodic
Mintezol	thiabendazole	anthelmintic
Mithracin	plicamycin	malignant hyper-calcaemia
Mitoxana	ifosfamide	cytotoxic
Mobiflex	tenoxicam	arthritis
Mobilan	indomethacin	arthritis

Proprietary Name	Approved Name	Main action or Indication
Modicate	fluphenazine	antipsychotic
Moditen	fluphenazine	schizophrenia
Modrasone	alclometasone	topical corticosteroid
Modrenal	trilostane	adrenal cortex inhibitor
Moduret 25	co-amilozide	diuretic
Moduretic	co-amilozide	diuretic
Mogadon	nitrazepam	hypnotic
Molipaxin	trazodone	antidepressant
Monaspor	cefsulodin	antibiotic
Monistat	miconazole	antifungal
Monit	isosorbide mononitrate	angina
Mono Cedocard	isosorbide mononitrate	angina
Monoclate-P	Factor VIII	haemophilia
Monocor	bisoprolol	beta-blocker
Monoparin	heparin	anticoagulant
Monotrim	trimethaprim	antibacterial
Monovent	terbutaline	bronchospasm
Motilium	domperidone	anti-emetic
Motrin	ibuprofen	arthritis
MST Continus	morphine	analgesic
Mucodyne	carbocisteine	mucolytic
Multiparin	heparin	anticoagulant
Myambutol	ethambutol	tuberculosis
Mycardol	pentaerythritol	coronary dilator
Mycifradin	neomycin	antibiotic
Mydriacyl	tropicamide	mydriatic
Mydrilate	cyclopentolate	mydriatic
Myleran	busulphan	cytotoxic
Myocrisin	sodium aurothiomalate	rheumatoid arthritis
Myotonine	bethanechol	cholinergic
Mysoline	primidone	epilepsy
Nacton	poldine	antispasmodic
Nalcrom	sodium cromoglycate	anti-allergic
Nalorex	naltrexone	opioid dependence
Naprosyn	naproxen	arthritis
Narcan	naloxone	narcotic antagonist
Nardil	phenelzine	antidepressant
Narphen	phenazocine	analgesic
Natrilix	indapamide	hypertension

Proprietary Name	Approved Name	Main action or Indication
Natulan	procarbazine	cytotoxic
Navidrex	cyclopenthiazide	diuretic
Naxogin	nimorazole	trichomoniasis
Nebcin	tobramycin	antibiotic
Negram	nalidixic acid	urinary antiseptic
Neo-Cytamen	hydroxocobalamin	anti-anaemic
Neo-Mercazole	carbimazole	thyrotoxicosis
Neo-Naclex	bendrofluazide	diuretic
Nephril	polythiazide	diuretic
Nerisone	diflucortolone	corticosteroid
Netillin	netilmicin	antibiotic
Neulactil	pericyazine	schizophrenia
Neupogen	filgrastim	neutropenia
Nidazol	metronidazole	trichomoniasis
Nimotop	nimodipine	subarachnoid haemorrhage
Nipride	sodium nitroprusside	hypertensive crisis
Nitoman	tetrabenazine	chorea
Nitrados	nitrazepam	hypnotic
Nitrocine	glyceryl trinitrate	angina
Nitrocontin Continus	glyceryl trinitrate	angina
Nitrolingual	glyceryl trinitrate	angina
Nitronal	glyceryl trinitrate	angina
Nivaquine	chloroquine	antimalarial
Nivemycin	neomycin	antibiotic
Nizoral	ketoconazole	antifungal
Nobrium	medazepam	antipsychotic
Noctec	chloral hydrate	hypnotic
Noltam	tamoxifen	cytotoxic
Nolvadex	tamoxifen	cytotoxic
Norcuron	vecuronium	muscle relaxant
Norditropin	somatropin	growth hormone
Nordox	doxycycline	antibiotic
Norflex	orphenadrine	muscle relaxant
Normetic	co-amilozide	diuretic
Normison	temazepam	hypnotic
Noroxin	norfloxacin	eye infections
Norval	mianserin	antidepressant
Novantrone	mitozantrone	cytotoxic
Noxyflex S	noxythiolin	antiseptic
Nozinan	methotrimeprazine	pain in terminal cancer

Proprietary Name	Approved Name	Main action or Indication
Nubain	nalbuphine	analgesic
Nystan	nystatin	antifungal
Ocusert Pilo	pilocarpine	glaucoma
Olbetam	acipimox	hyperlipidaemia
Omnopon	papaveretum	analgesic
Oncovin	vincristine	cytotoxic
One-alpha	alfacalcidol	vitamin D deficiency
Operidine	phenoperidine	analgesic
Ophthaine	proxymetacaine	corneal anaesthetic
Opilon	thymoxamine	vasodilator
Opticrom	sodium cromoglycate	allergic conjunctivitis
Optimine	azatadine	antihistamine
Orap	pimozide	schizophrenia
Orbenin	cloxacillin	antibiotic
Orimeten	aminoglutethimide	cytotoxic
Orudis	ketoprofen	arthritis
Oruvail	ketoprofen	arthritis
Otrivine	xylometazoline	nasal congestion
Ovex	mebendazole	anthelmintic
Oxanid	oxazepam	anxiolytic
Oxivent	oxitropium	bronchodilator
Palfium	dextromoramide	analgesic
Paludrine	proguanil	antimalarial
Panedeine	co-codamol	analgesic
Panadol	paracetamol	analgesic
Panmycin	tetracycline	antibiotic
Paracodol	co-codamol	analgesic
Parake	co-codamol	analgesic
Paramol	co-dydramol	analgesic
Paraplatin	carboplatin	cytotoxic
Parlodel	bromocriptine	lactation suppressant
Parmid	metoclopramide	anti-emetic
Parnate	tranylcypromine	antidepressant
Paroven	oxyrutins	varicose states
Parvolex	acetylcysteine	paracetamol overdose
Pavulon	pancuronium	muscle relaxant
Paxane	flurazepam	hypnotic
Pecram	aminophylline	bronchodilator
Penbritin	ampicillin	antibiotic
Pendramine	penicillamine	Wilson's disease
Penidural	benzathine penicillin	antibiotic

Proprietary Name	Approved Name	Main action or Indication
Pentacarinat	pentamidine	leishmaniasis
Pentasa	mesalazine	ulcerative colitis
Pentostam	sodium stibogluconate	leishmaniasis
Pepcid-PM	famotidine	H_2-blocker
Percutol	glyceryl trinitrate	angina
Perfan	enoximone	heart failure
Pergonal	menotrophin	hypogonadism
Periactin	cyproheptadine	antihistamine
Persantin	dipyridamole	angina
Pertofran	desipramine	antidepressant
Pevaryl	econazole	antifungal
Pharmorubicin	epirubicin	cytotoxic
Phasal	lithium carbonate	mania
Phenergan	promethazine	antihistamine
Phyllocontin Continus	aminophylline	bronchodilator
Physeptone	methadone	analgesic
Picolax	sodium picosulphate	laxative
Pimafucin	natamycin	antibiotic
Piportil	pipothiazine	antipsychotic
Pipril	piperacillin	antibiotic
Piptal	pipenzolate	antispasmodic
Piriton	chlorpheniramine	antihistamine
Plaquenil	hydroxy-chloroquine	antimalarial
Plendil	felodipine	calcium antagonist
Ponderax	fenfluramine	appetite suppressant
Pondocillin	pivampicillin	antibiotic
Ponstan	mefenamic acid	arthritis
Potaba	potassium p-aminobenzoate	scleroderma
Praxilene	naftidrofuryl	vasodilator
Precortisyl	prednisolone	corticosteroid
Predsol	prednisolone	corticosteroid
Preferid	budesonide	topical corticosteroid
Premarin	oestrogen	menopause
Prepidil	dinoprostone	cervical ripening
Prepulsid	cisapride	oesophageal reflux
Prescal	isradipine	calcium antagonist
Priadel	lithium carbonate	mania
Primacor	milrinone	servere heart failure

Proprietary Name	Approved Name	Main action or Indication
Primalan	mequitazine	antihistamine
Primaxin	imipenem	antibiotic
Primolut N	norethisterone	progestogen
Primperan	metoclopramide	anti-emetic
Pro-Banthine	propantheline	peptic ulcer
Profasi	gonadatrophin	infertility
Progesic	fenoprofen	arthritis
Proluton-Depot	hydroxy-progesterone	progestogen
Prominal	methylpheno-barbitone	epilepsy
Prondol	iprindole	antidepressant
Pronestyl	procainamide	cardiac arrhythmias
Propaderm	beclomethasone	topical corticosteroid
Propine	dipivefrin	glaucoma
Prostap	leuprorelin	prostatic carcinoma
Prostigmin	neostigmine	myasthenia
Prostin VR	alprostadil	maintenance of ductus arteriosus in neonates
Prothiaden	dothiepin	antidepressant
Pro-Vent	theophylline	bronchospasm
Provera	medroxy-progesterone	progestogen
Pro-Viron	mesterolone	androgen deficiency
Prozac	fluoxetine	antidepressant
Pulmadil	rimiterol	bronchospasm
Pulmicort	budesonide	rhinitis
Puri-Nethol	mercaptopurine	cytotoxic
Pyopen	carbenicillin	antibiotic
Quellada	lindane	pediculosis
Questran	cholestyramine	bile acid binder
Rapifen	alfentanyl	narcotic analgesic
Rastinon	tolbutamide	hypoglycaemic
Razoxin	razoxane	cytotoxic
Recormon	epoetin beta	anaemia in chronic renal failure
Redeptin	fluspirilene	schizophrenia
Redoxon	ascorbic acid	vitamin C deficiency
Refolinon	folinic acid	methotrexate antidote
Regaine	minoxidil	baldness
Rehibin	cyclofenil	infertility
Relefact	gonadorelin	test of pituitary function
Relifex	nabumetone	arthritis

Proprietary Name	Approved Name	Main action or Indication
Remnos	nitrazepam	hypnotic
Resonium A	exchange resin	hyperkalaemia
Restandol	testosterone	androgen deficiency
Retin A	tretinoin	acne
Retrovir	zidovudine	antiviral (AIDS)
Revanil	lysuride	parkinsonism
Rheomacrodex	dextran	blood volume expander
Rheumox	azapropazone	arthritis
Rhinocort	budesonide	rhinitis
Rumalgan	diclofenac	antirheumatic
Ridaura	auranofin	rheumatoid arthritis
Rifadin	rifampicin	tuberculosis
Rimactane	rifampicin	tuberculosis
Rinatec	ipatropium	rhinorrhoea
Rhinolast	azelastine	topical antihistamine
Rivotril	clonazepam	anticonvulsant
Roaccutane	isotretinoin	severe acne
Robaxin	methocarbamol	muscle relaxant
Robinul	glycopyrronium	peptic ulcer
Rocaltrol	calcitriol	vitamin D deficiency
Roccal	benzalkonium	antiseptic
Roferon-A	interferon	leukaemia
Rogitine	phentolamine	phaeochromocytoma
Rohypnol	flunitrazepam	hypnotic
Ronicol	nicotinyl alcohol	vasodilator
Roxiam	remoxide	schizophrenia
Rynacrom	sodium cromo-glycate	allergic rhinitis
Rythmodan	disopyramide	cardiac arrhythmias
Sabidal SR	theophylline	bronchospasm
Sabril	vigabatrin	anticonvulsant
Saizen	somatropin	growth hormone
Salazopyrin	sulphasalazine	ulcerative colitis
Salbulin	salbutamol	bronchodilator
Salbuvent	salbutamol	bronchodilator
Saluric	chlorothiazide	diuretic
Sandimmun	cyclosporin	immunosuppressant
Sandoglobulin	immunoglobulin	hepatitis
Sandostatin	octreotide	carcinoid syndrome
Sanomigran	pizotifen	migraine
Saventrine	isoprenaline	bronchospasm
Scoline	suxamethonium	muscle relaxant
Scopoderm TTS	hyoscine	motion sickness

Proprietary Name	Approved Name	Main action or Indication
Seconal	quinalbarbitone	hypnotic
Sectral	acebutolol	beta-blocker
Securon	verapamil	angina
Securopen	azlocillin	antibiotic
Selexidin	mecillinam	antibiotic
Selexid	pivmecillinam	antibiotic
Selsun	selenium sulphide	dandruff
Semprex	acrivastine	antihistamine
Septrin	co-trimoxazole	antibacterial
Serc	betahistine	Ménière's syndrome
Serenace	haloperidol	schizophrenia
Serevent	salmeterol	bronchospasm
Serophene	clomiphene	infertility
Seroxat	paroxetine	antidepressant
Serpasil	reserpine	hypertension
Sevredol	morphine	analgesic
Simplene	adrenaline	glaucoma
Sinemet	co-careldopa	parkinsonism
Sinequan	doxepin	antidepressant
Sinthrome	nicoumalone	anticoagulant
Sintisone	prednisolone	corticosteroid
Slo-Phyllin	theophylline	bronchodilator
Sloprolol	propranolol	beta-blocker
Slow-Pren	oxprenolol	beta-blocker
Slow-Trasicor	oxprenolol	beta-blocker
Soframycin	framycetin	antibiotic
Solu-Cortef	hydrocortisone	corticosteroid
Solu-Medrone	methylprednisolone	corticosteroid
Sominex	promethazine	mild hypnotic
Somnite	nitrazepam	hypnotic
Soneryl	butobarbitone	hypnotic
Sorbid SA	isosorbide dinitrate	angina
Sorbitrate	isosorbide dinitrate	angina
Sotacor	sotalol	beta-blocker
Sparine	promazine	antipsychotic
Spasmonal	alverine	antispasmodic
Spiroctan-M	canrenoate	diuretic
Spirolone	spironolactone	diuretic
Sporanox	itraconazole	antifungal
Stabillin V-K	penicillin V	antibiotic
Stafoxil	flucloxacillin	antibiotic
Staril	fosfinopril	ACE inhibitor
Stelazine	trifluoperazine	antipsychotic

Proprietary Name	Approved Name	Main action or Indication
Stemetil	prochlorperazine	anti-emetic
Stesolid	diazepam	anxiolytic
Stiedex	desoxymethasone	topical corticosteroid
Stiemycin	erythromycin	acne
Streptase	streptokinase	fibrinolytic
Stromba	stanozolol	anabolic steroid
Stugeron	cinnarizine	anti-emetic
Sublimaze	fentanyl	analgesic
Sulpitil	sulpiride	schizophrenia
Suprax	cefixime	antibiotic
Suprefact	busrelin	prostatic carcinoma
Surem	nitrazepam	hypnotic
Surgam	tiaprofenic acid	arthritis
Surmontil	trimipramine	antidepressant
Suscard Buccal	glyceryl trinitrate	angina
Sustac	glyceryl trinitrate	angina
Sustamycin	tetracycline	antibiotic
Sustanon	testosterone	androgen deficiency
Symmetrel	amantadine	parkinsonism
Synacthen	tetracosactrin	corticotrophin
Synalar	fluocinolone	topical corticosteroid
Synarel	nafarelin	endometriosis
Synflex	naproxen	arthritis
Synkavit	menadiol	hypoprothrombinaemia
Syntaris	flunisolide	local corticosteroid
Syntocinon	oxytocin	post-partum haemorrhage
Syntopressin	lypressin	diabetes insipidus
Syraprim	trimethoprim	antibacterial
Sytron	sodium iron edetate	anti-anaemic
Tachyrol	dihydrotachysterol	rickets
Tagamet	cimetidine	peptic ulcer
Talpen	talampicillin	antibiotic
Tambocor	flecainide	cardiac arrhythmias
Tamofen	tamoxifen	cytotoxic
Tanderil	oxphenbutazone	ocular inflammation
Targocid	teicoplanin	antibiotic
Tarivid	ofloxacin	urinary tract infections
Tavegil	clemastine	antihistamine
Teflox	temafloxacin	antibacterial
Tegretol	carbamazepine	anticonvulsant
Temgesic	buprenorphine	analgesic
Temopen	temocillin	antibiotic

Proprietary Name	Approved Name	Main action or Indication
Tenormin	atenolol	beta-blocker
Tensilon	edrophonium	diagnosis of myasthenia
Tenuate	diethylpropion	appetite suppressant
Teoptic	carteolol	glaucoma
Teronac	mazindol	appetite suppressant
Terramycin	oxytetracycline	antibiotic
Tertroxin	liothyronine	thyroid deficiency
Tetmosol	monosulfiram	scabies
Tetrabid	tetracycline	antibiotic
Tetrachel	tetracycline	antibiotic
Tetralysal	lymecycline	antibiotic
Theo-Dur	theophylline	bronchospasm
Thephorin	phenindamine	antihistamine
Ticar	ticarcillin	antibiotic
Tigason	etretinate	psoriasis
Tilade	neocromil	asthma
Tildiem	diltiazem	calcium antagonist
Timoptol	timolol	glaucoma
Tinset	oxatomide	antihistamine
Tobralex	tobramycin	eye infections
Tofranil	imipramine	antidepressant
Tolanase	tolazamide	hypoglycaemic
Tolectin	tolmetin	antirheumatic
Tonocard	tocainide	cardiac arrhythmias
Topicycline	tetracycline	acne
Topilar	fluclorolone	topical corticosteroid
Toradol	ketorolac	analgesic
Torecan	thiethylperazine	anti-emetic
Tracrium	atracurium	muscle relaxant
Trancopal	chlormezanone	anxiolytic
Trandate	labetalol	beta-blocker
Transiderm-Nitro	glyceryl trinitrate	angina
Tranxene	clorazepate	anxiolytic
Trasicor	oxprenolol	beta-blocker
Trasidex	co-prenozide	hypertension
Trasylol	aprotinin	pancreatitis
Travogyn	isoconazole	candidiasis
Traxam gel	felbinac	sprains
Tremonil	methixene	parkinsonism
Trental	oxpentifylline	vasodilator
Tridil	glyceryl trinitrate	angina
Triludan	terfenadine	antihistamine
Trimogal	trimethoprim	antibacterial

Proprietary Name	Approved Name	Main action or Indication
Trimopan	trimethoprim	antibacterial
Triperidol	trifluperidol	antipsychotic
Tritace	ramipril	ACE inhibitor
Trobicin	spectinomycin	antibiotic
Tropium	chlordiazepoxide	anxiety
Trosyl	tioconazole	antifungal
Tryptizol	amitriptyline	antidepressant
Tubarine	tubocurarine	muscle relaxant
Ubretid	dystigmine	urinary retention
Ukidan	urokinase	hyphaema; embolism
Ultralanum	fluocortolone	topical corticosteroid
Unasyn	sultamicin	antibiotic
Uniparin	heparin	anticoagulant
Uniphyllin Continus	theophylline	bronchospasm
Unisomnia	nitrazepam	hypnotic
Univer	verapamil	hypertension; angina
Uriben	nalidixic acid	urinary tract infections
Urispas	flavoxate	cystitis
Uromitexan	mesna	urotoxicity due to cyclophosphamide
Ursofalk	ursodeoxycholic acid	gallstones
Utinor	norfloxacin	urinary tract infections
Utovlan	ethisterone	progestogen
Uvistat	mexenone	sun screen
Valenac	diclofenac	arthritis
Valium	diazepam	anxiolytic; muscle relaxant
Vallergan	trimeprazine	sedative; pruritus
Valoid	cyclizine	anti-emetic
Vancocin	vancomycin	antibiotic
Vansil	oxamniquine	anthelmintic
Vascardin	isosorbide dinitrate	angina
Vascase	cilazapril	ACE inhibitor
Vasoxine	methoxamine	acute hypertension
Vasyrol	dipyridamole	arthritis
V-Cil-K	phenoxymethyl penicillin	antibiotic
Velbe	vinblastine	cytotoxic
Velosef	cephradine	antibiotic
Ventolin	salbutamol	bronchospasm
Vepesid	etoposide	cytotoxic

Proprietary Name	Approved Name	Main action or Indication
Vermox	mebendazole	anthelmintic
Vertigon	prochlorperazine	vertigo
Vibramycin	doxycycline	antibiotic
Videne	povidone-iodine	antiseptic
Vidopen	ampicillin	antibiotic
Virazid	tribavirin	antiviral
Virormone	testosterone	hypogonadism
Visclair	methylcysteine	mucolytic
Visken	pindolol	beta-blocker
Vivalan	viloxazine	antidepressant
Volital	pemoline	hyperkinaesia
Volmax	salbutamol	bronchodilator
Volramin	diclofenac	arthritis
Voltarol	diclofenac	antirheumatic
Welldorm	chloral hydrate	hypnotic
Wellferon	interferon	leukaemia
Xanax	alprazolam	anxiolytic
Xuret	metolazine	diuretic
Xylocaine	lignocaine	anaesthetic
Xylocard	lignocaine	cardiac arrhythmias
Yomesan	niclosamide	anthelmintic
Yutopar	ritodrine	premature labour
Zaditen	ketotifen	anti-asthmatic
Zadstat	metronidazole	trichomoniasis
Zantac	ranitidine	H_2-blocker
Zarontin	ethosuximide	anticonvulsant
Zavedos	idarubicin	cytotoxic
Zestril	lisinopril	ACE inhibitor
Zimovane	zopiclone	hypnotic
Zinacef	cefuroxime	antibiotic
Zinamide	pyrazinamide	tuberculosis
Zinnat	cefuroxime	antibiotic
Zirtek	cetirizine	antihistamine
Zithromax	azithromycin	antibiotic
Zocor	simvastatin	hyperlipidaemia
Zofran	ondansetron	anti-emetic
Zoladex	goserlin	prostatic carcinoma
Zovirax	acyclovir	antiviral
Zyloric	allopurinol	gout

Table 29. Cephalosporins

Orally active	Brand names	Daily dose range
cefaclor	Distaclor	750mg–4g
cefadroxil	Baxan	1–1.5g
cefixime	Suprax	200–400mg
cefuroxime	Zinnat	500mg–1g
cephalexin	Ceporex, Keftex	1–2g
cephadrine		1–2g
Cephalosporins given by IM or IV injection		**Daily dose range**
cefotaxime	Claforan	2–12g
cefoxitin	Mefoxin	3–12g
cefsulodin	Monospor	1–4g
ceftazidime	Fortum	1–6g
ceftizoxime	Cefizox	2–8g
cefuroxime	Zinacef	2–6g
cephalothin	Keflin	4–12g
cephamandole	Kefadol	2–12g
cephazolin	Kefzol	2–4g
cephradine	Velosef	2–8g

Table 30. Tetracyclines

Approved name	Brand name
chlortetracycline	Aureomycin
clomocycline	Megaclor
demeclocycline	Ledermycin
doxycycline	Vibramycin, Nordox
lymecycline	Tetralysal
minocycline	Minocin
oxytetracycline	Berkmycen, Imperacin, Terramycin, Unimycin

Table 31. Comparable doses of some corticosteroids

cortisone	25.0mg
hydrocortisone	20.0mg
prednisone	5.0mg
prednisolone	5.0mg
methylprednisolone	4.0mg
triamcinolone	4.0mg
dexamethasone	0.75mg
betamethasone	0.5mg

Table 32. Penicillins

Name	Main action/target	Administration/ injection
amoxycillin	broad-spectrum	oral, i.m.
ampicillin	broad-spectrum	oral, i.m., i.v.
azlocillin	antipseudomonal	i.v.
bacampicillin	ampicillin pro-drug	oral
benzylpenicillin	Gram-positive bacteria	i.m., i.v.
benethamine penicillin	long-acting penicillin	depot i.m.
benzathine penicillin	as benzylpenicillin	oral, i.m.
carbenicillin	antipseudomonal	i.m., i.v.
carfecillin	antipseudomonal	oral
cloxacillin } flucloxacillin }	penicillinase-producing staphylococci	oral, i.m., i.v.
mecillinam	Gram-negative and enterococcal bacteria	i.m., i.v.
methicillin	as cloxacillin	i.m., i.v.
mezlocillin	Gram-negative bacteria	i.m., i.v.
penicillin	see benzylpenicillin	
phenethicillin	as benzylpenicillin	oral
phenoxymethyl-penicillin	as benzylpenicillin	oral
piperacillin	broad-spectrum	i.m., i.v.
pivampicillin	ampicillin pro-drug	oral
pivmecillinam	mecillinam pro-drug	oral
procaine-penicillin	long-acting penicillin	i.m.
talampicillin	ampicillin pro-drug	oral
ticarcillin	antipseudomonal	oral

Intravenous additives

The slow intravenous infusion of drugs has, in some circumstances, certain advantages over other injection methods as a more even plasma level of the injected drug can be maintained over a longer period, and the disadvantages of a rapid bolus-type of injection are avoided. The method has its limitations as the addition of drugs to previously prepared intravenous fluids carries the risk of bacterial contamination, and strict aseptic precautions are essential during the preparation of any additive-containing intravenous fluid. In addition, incompatibility of the drug with the intravenous fluid may cause a loss of activity or, increase in toxicity, a risk that is increased if more than one drug is added to the infusion. Loss of activity may also occur because the stability of the drug is adversely influenced by dilution with the fluid and, in some cases, the pH of the infusion may play an important part as far as the stability and activity of the drug is concerned.

The preparation of additive-containing fluids is best carried out in the hospital pharmacy. If nurses prepare any such solutions on the ward or at the bedside, they should be fully acquainted with the techniques required and be aware of the risks involved. In all cases, complete mixing or solution of the drug in the fluid is essential before intravenous infusion is commenced, and the giving set should not be used for more than 24 hrs. Although the absence of any visual change in the appearance of the fluid is no guide to any loss of activity, any development of cloudiness in the solution, or a change of colour, is an indication that treatment should be stopped.

Intravenous additives are usually made to solutions of glucose 5%, or to sodium chloride solution 0.9%, although certain other fluids are also used, and any such extemporaneously prepared solution should be used as soon as possible, and only one bottle ought to be prepared at a time. Solutions containing sodium bicarbonate, mannitol, amino acids or blood products are not suitable vehicles for intravenous additives. The addition of drugs to intravenous fat emulsions is not recommended unless products specially formulated for the purpose are used. Such additions may break down the emulsion and cause embolism.

The intravenous infusion of drugs can be carried out by continuous or intermittent infusion. Some packs of continuous infusion fluids are designed to permit the addition of a drug in a way that reduces the risks of bacterial contamination, or the intermittent injection of a drug whilst the continuous infusion of the fluid is also taking place. With certain irritant cytotoxic drugs, the additive is not mixed with infusion fluid, but is injected via the tubing of a fast-running infusion fluid. Such a method permits the rapid dilution of the injected drug and so reduces the risks of vein irritation.

When a higher plasma level of a drug is required than can be obtained by continuous infusion, intermittent infusion is used, by which small volumes of about 100ml of the drug solution are infused over 30–60 min. The method is used for drugs that are relatively unstable in dilute solution, such as amoxycillin and some other antibiotics, and for drugs that are unsuitable for administration by drip infusion.

In Table 33, the abbreviation G refers to glucose 5%, and S to sodium 0.9%, although some other standard solutions such as Hartmann's Solution, or Ringer's Solution are used for additive-containing infusion fluids. In a few cases, Water for Injections (W) is preferred. CI refers to continuous intravenous infusion, I to intermittent infusion, and VDT to via drip tubing.

Table 33

Drug	Infusion fluid	Method of use
actinomycin D	G or S	VDT
acyclovir	G or S	I
alfentanil	G or S	CI, I
alprostadil	G or S	CI
amikacin	G or S	I
aminophylline	G or S	CI
amiodarone	G	CI, I
amoxycillin	G or S	I
amphotericin	G	CI (protect from light)
ampicillin	G or S	I
amsacrine	G	I
ancrod	S	CI
aprotinin	G or S	CI or VDT
atenolol	G or S	I
atracurium	G or S	CI

Drug	Infusion fluid	Method of use
azathioprine	G or S	VDT
azlocillin	G or S	I
aztreonam	G or S	I
betamethasone	G or S	CI or VDT
bleomycin	S	I
bumetanide	G or S	I
calcium gluconate	G or S	CI (not with sodium bicarbonate)
carbenicillin	G	I
carboplatin	G or S	CI
carmustine	G or S	I
cefotaxime	G or S	I
cefoxitin	G or S	I, VDT
cefsulodin	G or S	I, VDT
ceftazidime	G or S	I, VDT
ceftizoxime	G or S	CI, VDT
cefuroxime	G or S	I, VDT
cephalothin	G or S	I, VDT
cephamandole	G or S	I, VDT
cephazolin	G or S	I, VDT
cephradine	G or S	CI, I
chloramphenicol	G or S	I, VDT
cimetidine	G or S	CI, I
cisplatin	S	CI
clindamycin	G or S	CI, I
clomipramine	G or S	I
clonazepam	G or S	I
cloxacillin	G or S	I, VDT
co-amoxiclav	S	I
co-fluampicil	G or S	I
colistin	G or S	CI, I
co-trimoxazole	G or S	CI
cyclophosphamide	W	I, VDT
cyclosporin	G or S	CI
cytarabine	G or S	CI, I, VDT
dacarbazine	G or S	I
desferrioxamine	G or S	CI, I
dexamethasone	G or S	CI, I, VDT
diazepam	G or S	CI
digoxin	G or S	CI
dinoprost	G or S	CI
disodium etidronate	S	CI
disodium pamidronate	S or G	CI

Drug	Infusion fluid	Method of use
disopyramide	G or S	CI, I
dobutamine	G or S	CI (not with sodium bicarbonate)
dopamine	G or S	CI
doxorubicin	G or S	VDT
enoximone	S	CI, VDT
epirubicin	S	VDT
epoprostenol	S	I
erythromycin	G or S	CI, I
ethacrynic acid	G or S	VDT
etoposide	S	I
flecainide	G or S	CI, I
flucloxacillin	G or S	I, VDT
flumazanil	G or S	VDT
fluorouracil	G	CI, VDT
folinic acid	G or S	CI
frusemide	S	CI
fusidic acid	G or S	CI
ganciclovir	G or S	I
gentamicin	G or S	I, VDT
glyceryl trinitrate	G or S	CI
heparin	G or S	CI
hydralazine	S	CI
hydrocortisone	G or S	CI, I, VDT
ifosfamide	G or S	CI, I, VDT
imipenem	G or S	I
iron-dextran	G or S	I
isoprenaline	G or S	CI (well diluted)
isosorbide dinitrate	G or S	CI
isoxuprine	G or S	CI
kanamycin	G or S	I
labetalol	G or S	I
lignocaine	G or S	CI (well diluted)
mecillinam	G or S	I
melphalan	S	CI, VDT
mesna	G or S	CI, VDT
metaraminol	G or S	CI, VDT
methicillin	G or S	I, VDT
methocarbamol	G or S	I
methohexitone	G or S	I
methotrexate	G or S	CI, VDT (well diluted)
methyldopa	G	I
methylprednisolone	G or S	CI, I, VDT
metoclopramide	G or S	CI

Drug	Infusion fluid	Method of use
mexiletine	G or S	CI
mezlocillin	G or S	CI
miconazole	G or S	CI, I
mitozantrone	G or S	VDT
mustine	G or S	VDT
naloxone	G or S	CI
netilmicin	G or S	I, VDT
nimodipine	G or S	VDT
noradrenaline	G or S	CI (well diluted)
oxytocin	G or S	CI (well diluted)
pentamidine	G or S	I
phenoxybenzamine	S	I
phentolamine	G or S	I
phenylephrine	G or S	I
piperacillin	G or S	I
plicamycin	G	I (well diluted)
polymyxin B	G	CI
potassium chloride	G or S	CI (well diluted)
propofol	G or S	VDT
quinine dihydrochloride	S	CI
ranitidine	G or S	I
rifampicin	G or S	VDT
ritodrine	G or S	CI (well diluted)
salbutamol	G or S	CI
sodium nitroprusside	G	CI (well diluted; protect from light)
sodium valproate	G or S	CI, I
streptokinase	S	CI
sulphadiazine	S	CI
suxamethonium	G or S	CI
teicoplanin	G or S	I
terbutaline	G or S	CI
tetracosactrin	G or S	CI
tetracycline	G or S	CI
ticarcillin	G	I
tobramycin	G or S	I, VDT
tocainide	G or S	I
treosulfan	W	I
trimethoprim	G or S	VDT
urea	G	CI
urokinase	S	CI
vancomycin	G or S	I
vasopressin	G	I
vecuronium	G or S	I

Drug	Infusion fluid	Method of use
vidarabine	G or S	CI (well diluted)
vinblastine	S	VDT
vincristine	S	VDT
vindesine	G or S	VDT

Drugs and breast-feeding

Some drugs are known to be excreted to some extent in breast milk, and so should be avoided during breast-feeding, but in many cases information is scanty. Table 34 is only a general guide to the milk excretion of some standard drugs, and the omission of any drug does *not* imply that it is suitable for use during breast-feeding. Such use remains the responsibility of the prescriber. It might be wise to assume that if a drug of a certain class is listed, related drugs may have a similar pattern of excretion. If a drug is mentioned in more than one section, it may be that it is tolerated in low doses.

See table on pages 276–277.

Table 34. Drugs and breast-feeding

	Analgesics and anti-inflammatory drugs	**Antimicrobial agents**	**Cardiovascular drugs; anticoagulants**
Drugs that are contra-indicated	gold compounds phenylbutazone pencillamine indomethacin colchicine carisoprodol	chloramphenicol tetracyclines dapsone	amiodarone ergotamine phenindione
Drugs for use under control	salicylates	aminoglycosides antimalarials anthelmintics ethambutol isoniazid metronidazole nalidixic acid sulphonamides	anti-arrhythmics clonidine nicoumalone
Drugs usually considered safe in standard doses	codeine dextro-propoxyphene dihydrocodeine ibuprofen paracetamol pentazocine pethidine salicylates	penicillins cephalosporins erythromycin rifampicin metronidazole nitrofurantoin antifungal agents (except ketoconazole)	beta-blockers digoxin captopril heparin hydralazine methyldopa thiazide diuretics warfarin

	CNS depressants: antidepressants; anticonvulsants	**Drugs acting on the endocrine system**	**Miscellaneous**
Drugs that are contra-indicated	doxepin lithium salts	androgens oestrogens bromocriptine cyproterone carbimazole corticosteroids iodides	antineoplastics atropine calciferol vitamin A
Drugs for use under control	barbiturates carbamazepine benzodiazepines phenothiazines haloperidol phenobarbitone phenytoin primidone monoamine oxidase inhibitors	oestrogens thyroxine oral hypoglycaemics corticosteroids oral contraceptives	antihistamines amantadine aminophylline anthraquinone laxatives phenolphthalein cimetidine propantheline ranitidine sulphasalazine theophylline
Drugs usually considered safe in standard doses	benzodiazepines phenothiazines sodium valproate tricyclic antidepressants	progestogens ergometrine insulin	oral bronchodilators metoclopramide sodium cromoglycate vitamins folic acid

Oral contraceptives

The prevention of conception by the oral use of oestrogen–progestogen hormone products is a highly effective method of fertility control, but it is not free from risks. Oral contraceptives are contra-indicated when there is any history of thrombo-embolic disease, recurrent jaundice, liver disease, hyperlipidaemia, mammary and endometrial carcinoma and severe migraine. Side-effects include nausea, headache, weight gain, breast tenderness, depression, hypertension, benign hepatic tumours and reduced menstrual flow, which in some cases may amount to amenorrhoea. Care is necessary in hypertension, obesity, renal disease, varicose veins, asthma and epilepsy. Side-effects are considered to be more likely in women over the age of 35 and in cigarette smokers.

There is some evidence that the incidence of thrombo-embolic disease may be linked with the dose of oestrogen and, in general, those mixed products with a lower oestrogen content, yet which give adequate cycle control for the individual patient, should be used. On the other hand, those products with a higher dose of progestogen tend to reduce menstrual flow and increase weight gain.

Oral contraceptives fall into two groups, the oestrogen–progestogen group and the progestogen-only group. The former appear to act mainly by suppressing ovulation, but they may also influence the endometrium and hinder implantation. The are usually given in doses of one tablet from the 5th to the 25th day of the cycle, repeated after an interval of 7 days, but other dosage schemes are also in use. The so-called 'tri-phasic' products contain tablets of varying strengths of each constituent, and are designed to mimic the natural hormone cycle more closely than is possible with fixed dose products.

The progestogen-only products are considered to act by increasing the viscosity of cervical mucus, and so reduce sperm penetration. They are given in single daily doses, to be taken at the same time every day, and treatment must be continuous. Additional protection is necessary for the first 14 days, or if any dose is omitted. In general, they are considered less reliable than the mixed products, and they may cause menstrual irregularities.

Table 35 gives an indication of the range of products available.

Table 35

	Brand name	**Progestogen dose of product**
Mixed products containing 50μg of mestranol	Norinyl-1 Ortho-Novin 1/50	norethisterone 1mg
Mixed products containing 50μg of ethinyloestradiol	Minilyn Ovran	lynoestrenol 2.5mg levonorgestrel 250μg
Mixed products containing 35μg of ethinyloestradiol	Brevinor Neocon 1/35 Norimin Ovysmen	norethisterone 500μg norethisterone 1mg norethisterone 1mg norethisterone 500μg
Mixed products containing 30μg of ethinyloestradiol	Conova 30 Eugynon 30 Femodine Loestrin 30 Marvelon Microgynon 30 Minulet Ovran 30 Ovranette	ethynodiol 2mg levonorgestrel 250μg gestodene 75mg norethisterone 1.5mg desogestrel 150μg levonorgestrel 150μg gestodene 75mg levonorgestrel 250μg levonorgestrel 150μg
Mixed products containing 20μg of ethinyloestradiol	Loestrin 20 Mercilon	norethisterone 1mg desogestrel 150mg

Note: Logynon, Logynon ED, Binovum, Synaphase, Trinordiol, TriNovum and TriNovum ED are products containing tablets of different strengths of ethinyloestradiol and levonorgestrel, designed to give a phased hormonal effect.

Progestogen-only products	Femulen Micronor Microval Neogest Norgeston Noriday	ethynodiol 500μg norethisterone 350μg levonorgestrel 30μg norgesterel 75μg levonorgestrel 30μg norethisterone 350μg

Note: Depo-Provera is an injectable product containing medroxy-progesterone. A dose of 150mg by deep intra-muscular injection during the first 5 days of the cycle repeated after 3 months, has also been used as a contraceptive. Similarly, ethisterone oenanthate 200mg (Noristerat) may be given by deep intramuscular injection during the first 5 days of the cycle, and repeated once after 8 weeks.

Post-coital contraception has been obtained by the early administration of large doses of oestrogens, such as stilboestrol, in doses of 25mg twice a day for 5 days. Mixed products containing levonorgestrel 250μg and ethinyloestradiol 50μg (Schering PC4; Ovran; Eugynon 50) are now preferred, and treatment should be commenced within 72 hrs, followed by a second dose 12 hrs later. The risk of vomiting can be reduced by giving an anti-emetic such as prochlorperazine.

Weights and measures

Metric system

nanogram (ng) or 0.001μg
microgram (mcg or μg) or 0.001mg
milligram (mg) or 0.001g
centigram (cg) or 0.01g
decigram (dg) or 0.1g
gram (g) = 1000mg
(in prescriptions the abbreviation 'G' was formerly used, but is now obsolete.)
kilogram (kg) = 1000g

The metric measures of capacity which the nurse is likely to meet are the

millilitre (ml) which is approximately equal to the cubic centimetre (cc)
litre (l) = 1000ml

Imperial system

(No longer used for prescriptions)

ounce (oz)= 437.5 grains
pound (lb)= 16oz

ounce	= 480 minims
pint	= 20 fluid oz

Approximate metric and imperial equivalents

60mg	= 1 grain
1g	= 15 grains
28.4g	= 1oz
453g	= 1lb
1kg	= 2.2lb
63.5kg	= 10st
28.4ml	= 1floz
100ml	= 3.5floz
500ml	= 17.5floz
568ml	= 1pint
1000ml (1 litre)	= 35floz

Abbreviations used in prescriptions

The use of Latin abbreviations in prescription-writing is no longer recommended; the directions for use should be written in English, and in full. The use of some time-hallowed abbreviations still persist, and the following list is a selection of those terms that may be met with occasionally.

a.c.	*ante cibum*	before food
aq.	*aqua*	water
b.d.	*bis die*	twice a day
c.	*cum*	with
et	*et*	and
mitt.	*mitte*	send
o.n.	*omni nocte*	every night
p.c.	*post cibum*	after food
p.r.n.	*pro re nata*	occasionally
q.d.	*quater die*	four times a day
q.q.h.	*quarta quaque hora*	every four hours
q.s.	*quantum sufficiat*	sufficient
s.o.s.	*si opus sit*	when necessary
stat.	*statim*	at once
t.d.s.	*ter die sumendus*	to be taken three times a day
t.i.d.	*ter in die*	three times a day
ung.	*unguentum*	ointment

Notes: The abbreviations s.c., i.m. and i.v. refer to subcutaneous, intramuscular and intravenous injections. It is usually made clear when a drug must be given by *slow* intravenous *infusion*.

The doses of a few drugs are based on the skin area of the body expressed as square metres, abbreviated to m^2.